simply®

reflexology

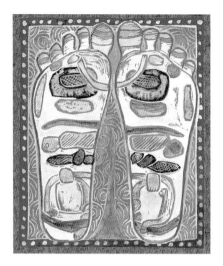

simply®

Reflexology

SONIA JONES

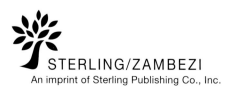

STERLING/ZAMBEZI

An imprint of Sterling Publishing Co., Inc.

New York / London
www.sterlingpublishing.com

STERLING and the distinctive Sterling logo are registered trademarks of Sterling Publishing Co., Inc.

Library of Congress Cataloging-in-Publication Data
Jones, Sonia, 1954-
Simply reflexology / Sonia Jones.
p. cm.
Includes index.
ISBA 978-1-4027-5455-5
1. Reflexology (Therapy) I. Title.
RM723.R43J66 2009
615.8'224—dc22
2008036754

2 4 6 8 10 9 7 5 3 1

Published by Sterling Publishing Co., Inc.
387 Park Avenue South, New York, NY 10016
Text © 2009 by Sonia Jones
Illustrations © Adam Reiti
Distributed in Canada by Sterling Publishing
c/o Canadian Manda Group, 165 Dufferin Street
Toronto, Ontario, Canada M6K 3H6
Published in the UK solely by Zambezi Publishing Ltd.
P.O. Box 221, Plymouth, PL2 2EQ
Distributed in Australia by Capricorn Link (Australia) Pty. Ltd.
P.O. Box 704, Windsor, NSW 2756, Australia

Printed in China
All rights reserved

Sterling ISBN 978-1-4027-5455-5
Zambezi ISBN 978-1-903065-64-8

For information about custom editions, special sales, premium and corporate purchases, please contact Sterling Special Sales Department at 800-805-5489 or specialsales@sterlingpublishing.com.

contents

introduction

Reflexology is a system of pressure and massage, a whole-body therapy that is applied through the feet and sometimes the hands, that works on many existing health conditions while also detecting potential future ailments. The treatment works with areas in the feet and hands that correspond to the body's tissues, glands, and organs, transported by a kind of subtle energy that takes the treatment to the area that needs to be healed. Reflexology can heal every part of the body, and it can heal the mind and soul as well, so it is a useful treatment for emotional problems in addition to health problems. Reflexology activates the self-healing response within the body, thus making this system a serious therapy in the health field.

Reflexology is not a new idea; it has been used for thousands of years. Here are some of the things that make reflexology so worthwhile:

- Anyone can learn it.
- It can be used on anyone from babies to the elderly.
- It doesn't require special equipment.
- It doesn't put anything into the body, so it is completely safe.
- You can do it anywhere and at any time.
- It is an extremely effective therapy.

Touch has always been a component of healing, and our basic instincts urge us to rub a sore area or to use pressure to relieve painful symptoms. When a child gets hurt, the child's mother invariably rubs and "kisses it better," and the child feels better as a result. Interestingly, parents often unconsciously massage their baby's feet while they hold the child on their laps, thus giving healing and comfort to the infant without realizing it.

A team of British doctors recently carried out a survey under scientific conditions to discover whether reflexology could help women with infertility problems. The results were poor, but during the experiment, it became clear that reflexology was extremely helpful to those who were sad or depressed. The doctors then widened the experiment to give reflexology to variety of men and women with different kinds of depression, and the results of this extended experiment were encouraging.

Reflexology has much more to offer than mere touch—and however relaxing and comforting it is, it also helps the mind and body to mend themselves. Many people who have cancer or who are postoperative seem to find their way to a reflexologist, and all of them find that reflexology helps them.

a note to the reader

You are strongly encouraged to find a book with detailed renderings of the human anatomy to use as reference. Having this material on hand as you peruse Chapters 7 through 10 will enhance your reading experience. You then will be able to envision exactly what systems or parts of the body will be affected by the reflexology treatment on different parts of the feet (or hands, as the case may be).

A thorough understanding of the material in Chapter 5, "The Zones," is essential to successful reflexology. You are urged to flag or otherwise highlight this chapter for easy accessibility, and refer to it repeatedly when exploring reflexology treatment.

Happy exploring!

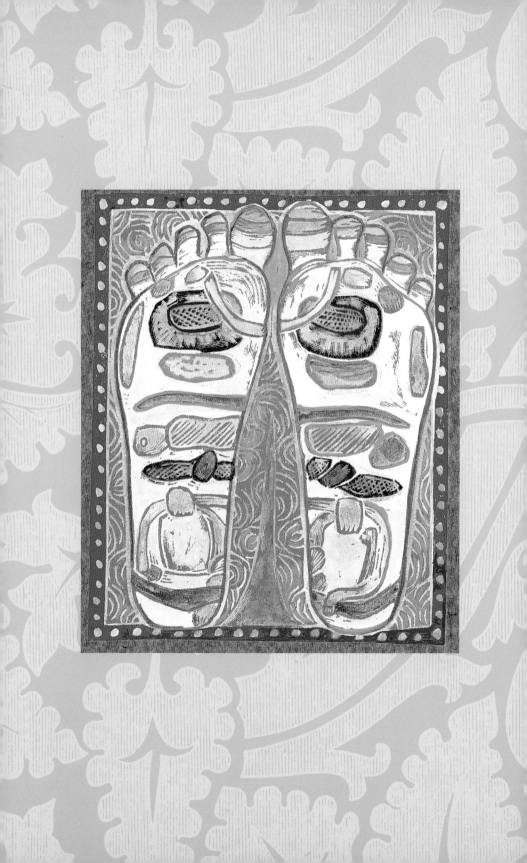

1

WHAT IS REFLEXOLOGY?

Our bodies constantly try to achieve homeostasis (a Greek word for "balance"), and medical textbooks devote many pages to explanations of the way that the body achieves this state. Our bodies regularly produce hormones and chemicals that speed up or slow down physical processes. When we get cold, our bodies shiver in an attempt to keep us warm; when we get hot, our sweat cools us down. Certain foods and drinks elevate our blood sugar levels, so the body responds by producing insulin, which brings the blood sugar levels down again. Some hormones break down calcium in our bones and others rebuild it. Reflexology stimulates responses in the body that help it to achieve homeostasis.

The feet and hands contain thousands of nerve endings, and stimulating these sensory nerve endings sends messages along the spinal cord to the brain. The areas of the hands or feet that are used in reflexology are called "reflex zones." Stimulation of these zones alerts the brain to potential problems and to the relevant areas of the body, and then the body itself decides whether to stimulate the affected area or to calm it down. Reflexology activates the body's own healing power, as do acupuncture and acupressure.

I have often been asked how I can bear to touch people's feet. I find nothing wrong with feet as long as they are clean. We don't mind touching people's hands, but hands touch door handles, railings, buttons on elevators, and so on, while feet stay inside clean socks all day. Most people never touch another person's feet, and they rarely allow others to touch their feet. Yet reflexology feels so wonderful—it's a real treat! Even a short foot massage can ease away a stressful day and make you feel less tired. Everyone loves a foot massage.

The second thing people say is that their feet are far too ticklish to be treated, but during the many years that I have practiced reflexology, this has never been a problem. The feet are handled in such a way that even the most sensitive people do not experience any problem at all.

Studies have shown that those who incorporate some fulfilling activities into their lives, such as meditation or an absorbing hobby, or who give some form of treatment to others are healthier, happier, and more positive and effective in all areas of their lives.

Tip: Though reflexology does not treat specific diseases, it does bring about a change in the body that enables it to heal itself.

A BRIEF HISTORY OF REFLEXOLOGY

Reflexology goes back thousands of years—to ancient Egypt, China, and many other ancient cultures. Many ancient texts have been found on the subject of healing through the hands and feet. Just like acupuncture, reflexology has stood the test of time.

Around the beginning of the twentieth century, Dr. William Fitzgerald developed the modern form of reflexology, which he called "zone therapy." He explained the concept of parts of the body corresponding to other parts of the body. To the surprise of those who observed his methods, he provided proof by applying pressure to an area of a patient's hand and showing that the corresponding area in the body became anesthetized: He stuck a pin into a patient's cheek without causing the patient any pain, while applying pressure on the area of the hand that corresponded to the face.

In the 1930s, a physiotherapist named Eunice Ingram used zone therapy on her patients with great success. It came to her attention that the zones that run throughout the body could be accessed anywhere along the zone, but she discovered that the feet were the most sensitive and the most responsive of the areas that run along the zones.

After much work and research, Eunice Ingram had mapped out on the feet the pressure points that corresponded to the whole body. Working on different areas on the feet with alternating pressure, she soon discovered that this treatment had far-reaching therapeutic consequences. Not long after this, zone therapy became known as reflexology.

Since Fitzgerald's and Ingram's days, the research has continued, and reflexology has progressed from strength to strength. It was in the mid-1980s that reflexology really took off, and since then it has grown tremendously all around the world. Now nearly everyone has heard about reflexology and knows that it is a treatment applied mainly to the feet that brings about a change in the whole body.

HOLISTIC MEDICINE

Reflexology is truly a holistic treatment; it falls under the umbrella term "alternative or complementary medicine." Alternative medicine is an alternative to conventional medicine, and the word "complementary" suggests something that can complement or work alongside conventional medicine. Both terms apply to reflexology. Holistic medicine is a system of health care that is completely different in its philosophy, approach, and practice from conventional medicine, which is also known as allopathic medicine. In holistic medicine a person is viewed as a physical, psychological, and emotional being, with a complete mind, body, and soul connection. Holistic medicine gives the body what it needs to heal itself naturally.

The body will always endeavor to heal itself, which means that a cut will heal and a broken bone will mend. Holistic implies "the whole," which in this case means "the whole person." Like a watch, "the whole" needs to be in good working order for it to keep good time. All the components of the body need to be working well for the body to be in balance. Reflexology is extremely effective at encouraging the body to ensure that all the parts are in good working order; therefore, it encourages balance. As all systems in the body are completely interrelated, only one part needs to be slightly out of balance for problems to arise in other systems of the body. If left untreated, these can become chronic problems.

In conventional medicine, the human body is viewed very differently, and in ever-smaller components. You might have a nasal problem that makes it impossible to breathe through your nose or to smell or taste your food properly. The conventional solution might be to prescribe antihistamine medication. The antihistamine will provide relief, but its effects are temporary. From a holistic point of view, it is important to find the cause of the congestion and to discover why the body is producing too much or too little mucus. More often than not, medicine suppresses a part of the body or a function, and that gives the appearance of balance. Pain is another example, as chronic pain from neck aches, backaches, and frequent headaches is treated with painkillers, which work quickly and effectively. However, once their effect wears off, the headache returns and more medication is needed. Rather than continue this cycle, the patient could take a different approach to find out why he or she is suffering from chronic headaches in the first place.

Most people prefer the term "complementary medicine" to "holistic medicine" because most people opt for both forms of medicine and believe that they complement each other. Many doctors in group practice now have alternative practitioners working in or near their practices, thus proving that there is a place for both types of healing.

Reflexology is often available at sports clubs, activity cen-
ters, hotels with spas and sports facilities, health farms, and
country clubs. People see it as a mainstream treatment
rather than something about which to be fearful, suspicious,
or cautious.

Reflexology is useful for anybody who is taking medicines,
because the treatment doesn't introduce another product
into the body in the way that aromatherapy and herbal treatments do. Herbs and essential oils may block or interfere
with the action of important medical drugs, but reflexology
should be safe to use under most circumstances, including
when the client is taking medication.

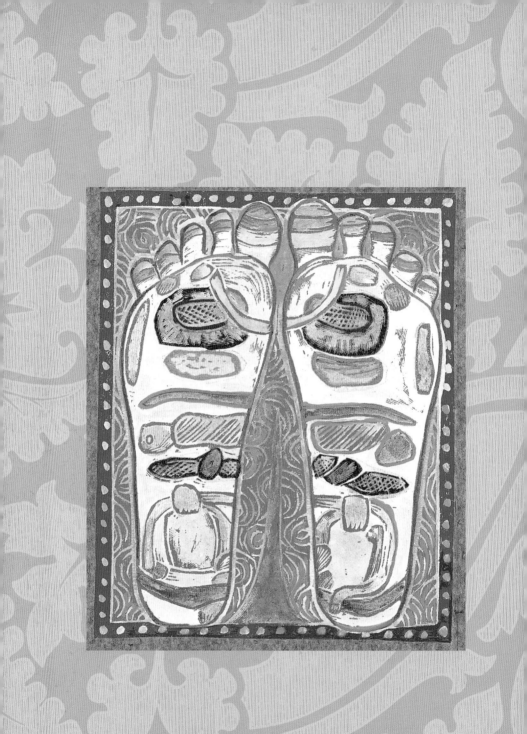

2

THE BENEFITS OF REFLEXOLOGY

It may surprise you to discover how far-reaching the benefits of reflexology can be. Not only is it a truly holistic treatment, but it is also an extremely pleasant experience. People get hooked on the good experience of the treatment and the health benefits that they gain from it.

A STRESS BUSTER

Stress is a fact of life—none of us can escape it—but it is not the stress that is the problem so much as the way we perceive it and the way we handle it. We are all different, and some people handle stress better than others, but it's also true that there are good and bad stresses. For instance, performing in your amateur dramatic society is stressful in an exhilarating way, but worry, frustration, overwork, relationship difficulties, and money concerns are harmful stresses. As they mount up and our defenses sink, we become more susceptible to illnesses.

So the answer is to find ways of coping with stress and to give the body the necessary tools to cope with these life stresses. Reflexology has been proved over the years to be a really good therapy for coping with stress. If you have reflexology on a regular basis, while at the same time figuring out how you can solve some of your problems and put them into perspective, this can be a lifesaver. Ask yourself whether you work too many hours. How do you feel about your job? Do you have meaningful relationships? Do you have a hobby, interests, and friends that help you to relieve your stress? How is your diet? Some types of food and drink can be extremely stressful to the body and can cause a real sense of anxiety.

The way we handle stress has a huge bearing on the way we age. During times of worry, our stress hormone levels rise; in young people the levels soon drop back down again, but in older people these higher levels can take days to drop. These prolonged periods when high levels of stress hormones are circulating in our systems eventually have a negative affect on our overall health and well-being. So how can we help to lower our stress hormone levels? One way is to have regular treatments of reflexology.

REFLEXOLOGY IMPROVES QUALITY OF SLEEP

If we can't get a good night's sleep, the world starts to look like a very different place. It becomes harder to cope with everyday life. Relationships become difficult because our nerves are frayed, and everything seems just a little more irritating. Children are noisier, the boss is more demanding than ever, and worries are magnified.

Reflexology works on a deep level to bring about a real sense of peace, and most people say they sleep much better during periods of treatment. The body can cope with the occasional restless night or even an odd late night, but when this disruptive sleep pattern becomes a regular occurrence, it affects long-term health in a negative way. Sleeping well is extremely important for deep healing and regeneration.

During restful, rejuvenating sleep, the body produces human growth hormone, sometimes called "the youth hormone." During sound sleep, our stress hormone levels fall, which is important to our overall well-being and long-term health. The world looks so much better after a good night's sleep! Reflexology enhances the quality of our sleep, thus slowing down the aging process and reducing the level of our stress hormones.

Some of the things we ingest can affect our sleep negatively as well. Drinking alcohol in the evening on a regular basis will initially make you drowsy, but later your body experiences a burst of norepinephrine, a stimulant that disturbs sleep and causes the body to feel below par. Coffee contains caffeine, a stimulant that interferes with your quality of sleep and elevates your stress hormones.

Outside events also can make it hard to sleep. An obvious one is a new baby, but living in a noisy part of town or not having curtains thick enough to keep the room dark can also disrupt sleep. Sometimes, for whatever reason, your mind refuses to switch off. An uncomfortable bed or a pillow that is wrong for your sleeping position won't help, either, but in all cases, reflexology can help you to relax and get a better night's sleep.

REFLEXOLOGY IMPROVES CIRCULATION

The circulation carries the blood around the body. The blood transports oxygen and nutrients to nourish the cells and removes carbon dioxide and debris for processing by the liver and kidneys, so anything that improves the circulation will improve overall health. The cells make up tissue that forms the arteries, heart, bones, liver, skin, and so much more. The blood vessels contract and relax, enabling the blood to reach every outpost in the body. Stress, fatigue, and illness can affect this flow, as the blood vessels become constricted, which hinders the flow of blood, especially to the brain and extremities. If we improve our circulation, we improve the function of every cell, and this improves everything from our stamina to our state of mind.

REFLEXOLOGY HELPS TO CHARGE OUR BATTERIES

Wouldn't we all like more energy? I have come across people in their seventies and eighties who have loads of energy and others in their thirties who struggle to keep up. Feeling more energetic gives us a zest for life; it makes our daily tasks easier and more enjoyable. This energy can be described as a life force. I am sure you have met people who are full of this life force. The Chinese call this energy "chi," and chi needs to flow unimpeded around the whole body. If this chi, or life force, becomes blocked, we feel listless and may even experience pain. Reflexology opens up the energy pathways, enabling a free flow of this energy throughout the body.

You shouldn't confuse zest for life with the hyperactive type of energy that can be unsettling. That is a false energy and will deplete you in the long run. Other forms of energy come from such things as sugar and caffeine, which pick you up quickly but don't give real, lasting energy. You may even end up unable to function properly without stimulants. These stimulants cause your organs a huge amount of stress and eventually leave you even more depleted. If you are one of those people who need a cup of coffee or tea or a sugary refined starch breakfast before you can get going in the morning, your chi is depleted. After a night's sleep we should be refreshed and renewed, without the need for caffeine or sugar.

REFLEXOLOGY HELPS US TO DETOX

The lymphatic system is one of our bodies' major detoxifying networks. The lymphatic system is susceptible to sluggishness because of the very nature of its design and because of our modern lifestyles. Our blood circulation has a pump, the heart, and that ensures efficient delivery of blood around our bodies. The lymphatic system is very different, as it relies on muscle movement to convey lymph around the body. Nowadays so many people lead sedentary lives—they sit at work, drive everywhere, watch television, go to the movies, a bar, or a restaurant, and in fact do very little other than sit in one place or another. This isn't an ideal situation for our lymphatic system, and if we couple that scenario with a poor diet, the lymphatic system can quite easily get clogged up or become extremely sluggish. This can lead to a variety of health conditions, as well as more superficial problems such as cellulite. When the lymphatic system becomes compromised, other systems of detoxification have more work than would otherwise be expected of them, and this puts extra strain on them. Reflexology helps to move the lymph, encouraging it to be more efficient, helping to take the workload off the organs of elimination, such as the liver, kidneys, lungs, bowels, and skin. Reflexology also helps these organs, not just the lymphatic system, to perform a better job.

REFLEXOLOGY ENCOURAGES PREVENTION

As the saying goes, an ounce of prevention is worth a pound of cure. We have our cars serviced on a regular basis, and this should also be true for ourselves. We should take prevention seriously and have regular treatments to keep us balanced. Some people tell me that their prevention strategy is to have regular blood tests—to measure cholesterol levels, blood pressure, blood glucose, triglycerides, and so on. This is monitoring rather than prevention, though, and these tests might even be a bit too late, as they will show when something has already gone wrong. In holistic medicine, we can spot in advance an organ or system that is struggling, and we can advise and help our clients to lead a healthier lifestyle, which includes treatments such as reflexology.

PART OF THE WHOLE

The feet contain information about the whole body, as do the hands, face, ears, tongue, spine, and iris (in the eye). Some acupuncturists treat only the ears (a treatment called "auricular acupuncture") but still achieve amazing results. Another technique is iridology, in which reading the iris can reveal what is happening within the whole body; after the reading, the iridologist must decide on the course of treatment needed. In reflexology, the reflexologist can read the feet, but he or she can also work on the whole system at the same time. In other words, the treatment is carried out on the entire body in a totally holistic way. This treatment signals the body to decide for itself the course of action that it needs for healing. For instance, the client may have a hormone imbalance, and by working the whole body via the feet (or hands), the reflexologist activates the body into balancing the endocrine system. Only the body can possibly know the delicate formula needed for a harmonious hormone symphony.

Reflexology works on the emotional, physical, and spiritual levels. Some people cry during treatment because it releases emotional tension or blockage, but in my experience crying is not a common reaction. I have often seen people find the strength and courage to make necessary life-changing decisions after a course of treatment. Reflexology works on many different levels, but all are positive healing responses. The body never does anything detrimental to itself; it doesn't harm itself. We are the ones who harm our bodies, so in a way, we are our own worst enemies. We often treat our pets better than we do ourselves.

As well as being a reflexologist, I am a naturopath and nutritional therapist, so I firmly believe, through firsthand experience, that we are what we eat. However, I also firmly believe that we are what we do. Over the years we adopt behavior patterns that are detrimental to our health and well-being, and even our posture can cause us pain.

Another saying proclaims that "You are what you think." I once heard a related, old-fashioned saying that states, "By the time you reach your old age, you have the face you deserve." I love that saying. Look at an old person's face and you might see, for instance, a permanent frown, scowl, or grimace, radiating anger, pain, and irritation. But look at another old person's face and you might see a smile etched into it radiating kindness, calm, and patience. Like our faces, our bodies also eventually reflect our lifestyles, the food and drinks we decide to consume, the thoughts we choose to think, and the behavioral patterns (physical and emotional) we continue to adopt. A person who eats well, who is happy, active, confident, and successful (success means something different to everyone), and who is in a good relationship will suffer fewer chronic illnesses, be less susceptible to viruses, and have far fewer aches and pains than a person who is less well adjusted. An individual who chooses a decent lifestyle that includes good nutrition and reasonable activity, and who nurtures valuable relationships and breaks off those that create unhappiness, will have good health. These people still experience stress in their lives, but they will see their cups as half full as opposed to half empty. Reflexology can help, sometimes by giving an individual the impetus to make necessary changes to improve his or her life. Reflexology helps to balance your brain chemistry and to balance your hormones; it encourages better sleep, gives you more energy, and generally makes you more optimistic.

Giving a treatment to others can also be very beneficial to your overall health and well-being, as it will make you more relaxed. As you use your fingers and thumbs, you stimulate the tips of your fingers, the ends of the meridians and acupuncture points. (Meridians are invisible or "subtle" lines that run through the body, carrying energy along their length. Acupuncturists and acupressurists work on these points to send healing to the appropriate body areas.) There is something very fulfilling about helping people, whether they are your family and friends or strangers. There is also the added benefit of learning something new, which has been proved to be good for both client and practitioner.

BABIES AND CHILDREN

It is very important for those who treat children with reflexology to recognize when a child should be referred to a doctor. They say that mothers know instinctively when something is wrong with their children and when it's bad enough to see or call the doctor, so if you are a mother, follow your instincts.

Babies respond extremely well to reflexology—they really like it. Very gently rubbing their fingers and toes can work wonders. This will help a lot for babies when they are teething, for example, as it eases their pain so they can sleep better; therefore, it will also do wonders for the quality of your sleep!

If your baby is fretful or if she or he has an earache, very gently caress the area of the foot beneath the instep in a circular motion; this will help to calm the baby and it will help the healing process. The pressure used on your baby's hands and feet should be a light caressing or stroking rather than pressing.

Children love having their hands and feet touched and rubbed. As children get older, you can use the caterpillar movement on their feet—that is, a walking movement with the fingers and thumbs rather than a rub—but with much less pressure than you would use on adult feet and hands. In this way, children can reap all the same benefits that adults who receive reflexology do.

Children often suffer from unexplained tummy upsets that might be caused by nerves or anxiety. Gently stroke the sole of the foot under the instep to calm their anxieties and make the "butterflies" go away.

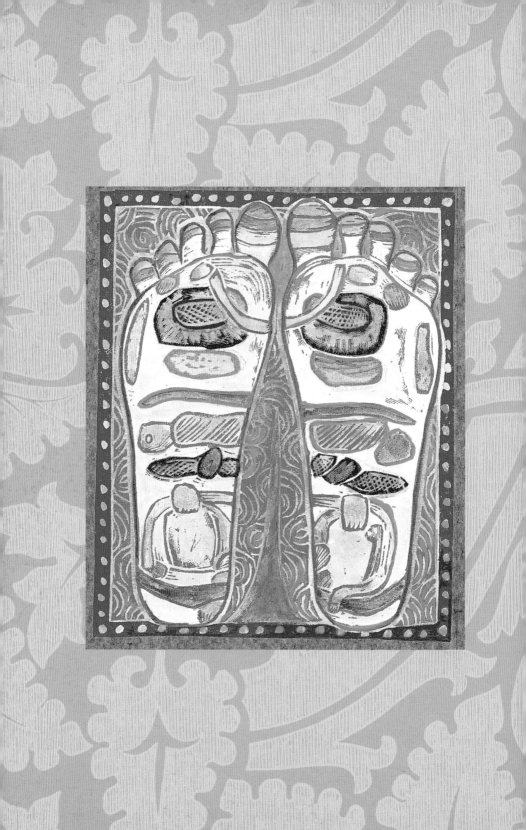

3

THE HEALING CRISIS

Not everyone suffers a "healing crisis" after treatment—in fact, most don't—but for those who do, here is what happens.

Some people find that after a full body massage, for example, their necks and shoulders hurt, or they feel worse rather than better. Others get headaches. These reactions are due to the muscles releasing stored toxins. This can happen after a reflexology session, although it doesn't happen often, and if it does occur, it goes away quickly. People usually feel much better after a reflexology treatment, so if you are one of the vast majority of people who do not experience a healing crisis, don't feel that you have been shortchanged. It doesn't mean that the healing method hasn't worked; your body is still striving for balance and the healing process has still been activated, regardless of the lack of a healing crisis.

Among those who do suffer a reaction after a reflexology session, colds are very common. I have come across a lot of people over the years who have come down with a heavy cold after a few sessions of reflexology. This is the body's way of releasing stored up toxicity and emotions. Even when people are warned about this potential healing crisis, they often don't deal with it properly. They have become so accustomed to taking medication for colds over the years that they don't realize that the cold itself is part of the healing process and treating it in this way works against the reflexology treatment.

Here are other reactions that some people may experience after treatments:

- Slightly worse symptoms for twenty-four hours after treatment
- Loads of energy
- Pimples
- Fatigue for a few days—needing lots of sleep
- Better moods
- Less pain
- More mobility
- A next menstrual period that may be heavier than usual
- A headache that lasts for a few hours
- Feeling more relaxed

DURING A TREATMENT

Here are some things that you may experience during a reflexology treatment. The release of emotions is quite common, and everyone expresses this in different ways.

- Crying
- Laughing
- Sweating
- Coughing
- Sighing
- Erection
- Twitching
- Sudden cramp
- Fatigue
- Headache
- Passing gas

- Burping
- Gurgling
- Relaxing

After a treatment, it is very important to drink plenty of water throughout the rest of the day. This water should not be cold from the fridge and should not contain ice; it should be at room temperature. Add some fresh lemon juice to help the body remove toxins. A reflexology treatment stirs up toxins, so it is important to give the system assistance to ensure that these toxins are flushed out. This will automatically reduce the likelihood of suffering a healing crisis. You may prefer to drink a variety of weak herbal teas (without sugar or milk) such as peppermint, chamomile, boldo, linden, pau d'arco, and raspberry leaf; there are many others to choose from as well. Make a pot of tea using the tea in its loose-leaf form, and take time out.

CONTRAINDICATIONS

Reflexology treatment should not be given in the presence of any of the following:

- Diabetes (hand reflexology is good, but foot reflexology might be harmful)
- Pregnancy, especially if there is a history of miscarriage
- A pacemaker
- A contagious disease
- An open sore or sore skin
- A new injury (external or internal)

- An old injury if there is any discomfort
- An area of broken veins (the area will be dark red with stagnant blood)
- Areas with fluid retention
- Varicose veins

If you have any doubts, even if none of the above conditions are present, do not perform a reflexology treatment.

Never persuade anyone to have a reflexology treatment or any other kind of treatment against his or her will, even if you are certain that it would help that person. If someone doesn't want to be treated, it's always better to leave him or her alone.

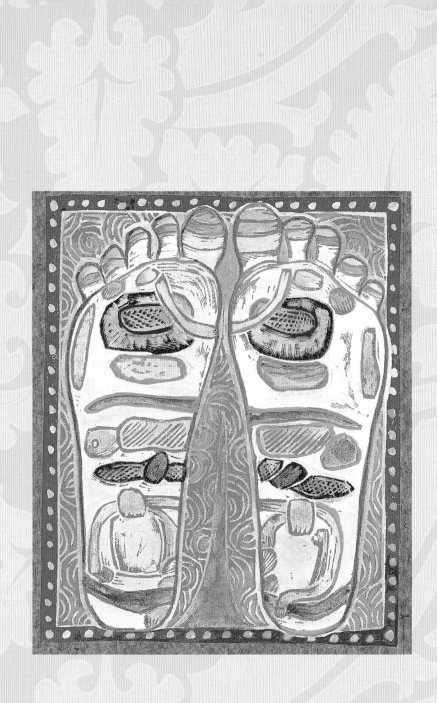

4

READING THE FEET

CONDITIONS THAT NEED SPECIAL CONSIDERATION

Gout affects mostly the big toes, but it can occasionally affect the ankles and knees. It is extremely painful; the big toe swells up, becomes very inflamed, turns red, and throbs. The condition affects men more than women and is the consequence of a buildup of uric acid in the blood. This is most often due to the body's inability to metabolize nitrogen-containing compounds properly. These nitrogens are known as purines, and they are found in abundance in a typical Western diet. Reflexology is effective in treating this condition, as the treatment encourages the organs of elimination and detoxification to work more efficiently. Treatment may have to wait until the toe is less painful and inflamed, however, and dietary changes should be made. If left untreated, gout can cause joint deformities. If it isn't wise to treat the feet, you can give reflexology to the hands instead.

Diabetics need to take their condition seriously and control their blood sugar levels, be it naturally or pharmaceutically. If the person to whom you are giving reflexology has diabetes, you need to be extra careful to avoid scratching him or her, as diabetes makes people very susceptible to infections and their wounds heal very slowly. Their feet can be extra-sensitive or not sensitive enough for the patient to know when they are being damaged. More often than not they are not sensitive enough due to nerve damage. In very extreme cases gangrene can set in, but this is not common. If in doubt, treat a diabetic's hands, because they tend to have better circulation and more feeling in them.

Lack of circulation is a common condition, and sufferers have cold, pale feet. The circulation struggles to get enough blood—and hence enough oxygen and nutrients—to the extremities. This problem can also affect the brain, as that, too, needs a healthy blood supply. Reflexology will enhance the whole circulatory system, ensuring a better supply of oxygen and nutrients to all parts of the body. Better circulation means that more oxygen and nutrients reach the heart muscle, which in turn improves blood flow around the body.

Spider veins are a common condition as we age; this condition is most often seen around the insides of the feet under the anklebones. When doing reflexology, be careful around these areas and use very gentle pressure, as the veins can break.

Chilblains are an inflammation of the small blood vessels in the skin in response to cold weather. This condition results in red, swollen skin usually on the toes and fingers, but sometimes on the ears and face. Chilblains appear several hours after the areas have been exposed to the cold and result in an itching and burning sensation. In some cases chilblains can develop into blisters and even open sores. Never perform reflexology on any broken, sore, or blistered skin. When temperatures drop, the affected areas should be kept warm, but if the areas get cold, it is very important to rewarm them very slowly. Never put hands affected with chilblains on radiators or into hot water. When the chilblains are in remission, regular reflexology treatments should be given because they will improve the condition by improving the body's circulation in general.

Edema is a condition in which the sufferer has an accumulation of fluid in the tissue, often in the ankles and feet. It is obvious to the naked eye that these areas are very swollen; they can sometimes be painful to the touch. Shoes can be painful to wear. Foot reflexology can be painful in these cases as well, so treat the hands, and later when the condition improves, start treating the feet. Make sure the person is not dehydrated. Many people drink very little, and this becomes very evident with people with edema, because they think that if they drink water their condition will be made worse. This is not the case, and more often than not, drinking water helps the condition. Coffee and soft drinks are dehydrating and should be avoided. Check with the person with edema to determine whether he or she has seen a doctor about the problem, as edema can denote a heart condition.

Athlete's foot is a fungal infection that appears between the toes, and it seems to affect men more than women. It is a systemic problem that needs to be treated with herbal remedies and a change in diet. For this condition it is advisable to do reflexology on the hands. The therapy will help to strengthen the immune system, which in turn helps the body to fight this condition.

Tip: Reflexology is not a tool for diagnosis, but with some observation skills, you can discover whether the body is struggling and if it is in need of some help. The signs we observe are the body's way of telling us something is out of balance. Just like pain, any disorder is a warning signal. Reflexology, because it is a holistic treatment, gives the body the necessary impetus to make positive changes for itself.

The color of the feet is a good place to start your observation. Are the feet pale all over? Are they cold to the touch? If the answer is yes, the person's circulation is not as good as it could or should be. Is there paleness in just parts of the feet? If a part of a foot is pale, see which reflex it represents, as this will show what is making the client unwell.

Red patches on the feet can reveal problems with the parts of the body that correspond to the relevant reflex zones.

Hard skin found on different parts of the feet relates to the corresponding part of the body. About twenty-five years ago I gave up smoking, at a time before I really knew much about reflexology. In those days I had a lot of hard skin on the balls of my feet that often caused me discomfort, but I just assumed it was from wearing high heels. Some years later I started to learn about reflexology, and it suddenly occurred to me that all the hard skin that had built up was gone! This hard skin buildup had been under the ball of my foot, which relates to the lung reflex area. Now that my health has improved, I still wear high heels but I no longer have the hard skin problem.

The area of the toes around the joints is associated with parts of the body that include the eyes, ears, sinuses, and neck, so crooked or bent toes can indicate a problem in one or more of these areas. Crooked toes can also indicate a nervous type of person or someone who is under a lot of stress.

Toes that point up can reveal a person who is energetic and who has a large appetite. That grand appetite might be for food or it could be for life in general.

Fungus under the toenail or between the toes is a systemic problem (this means that the problem is in the whole body, not just the toes—it's in the system in general). Tea tree essential oil can do wonders on a superficial level, but the underlying cause needs to be addressed. It is possible this person has had too many antibiotics, creating a systemic imbalance, in which case he or she needs to take an intensive course of probiotics, which can be found in any good health store. Alternatively, this person may eat too many sugary or refined foods, encouraging the wrong bowel flora, therefore allowing a fungal infection to take over. The person's immune system may have become run down, allowing this opportunistic fungal infection to take hold. Reflexology, along with a reduction of sugar and refined foods and a supplement of probiotics, will strengthen the immune system and change the bowel flora.

There are several possible reasons for dry skin:

1 Dehydration is a widespread problem these days. Too many people drink dehydrating fluids such as coffee, soft drinks, and so on. Most people do not drink enough water or hydrating fluids.
2. Deficiencies of essential fatty acids are also a common problem these days, as most people eat the wrong sorts of fats or have become "fat phobic" and don't eat enough fat. Essential fatty

acids come from oily fish, raw nuts and seeds, and supplements such as evening primrose oil, flaxseed oil, and fish oil capsules.

3. A digestive problem may be present; it may be that food is not being broken down properly or nutrients are not being absorbed properly.

Nails can reveal much about your general health:

1. Vertical ridges show that the liver is being overworked.
2. Concave nails denote anemia or low blood pressure.
3. Nails that rise from the finger suggest lung problems.
4. Grooves can show poor nutrient absorption or arthritis.
5. Bumps and ridges denote imbalance in the intestines, heart trouble, or severe stress.
6. Dark red to purple color shows too much fat and sugar in the blood.
7. Pale nails show anemia, while a blue color suggests heart problems.
8. Split, cracking nails show poor nutrition.

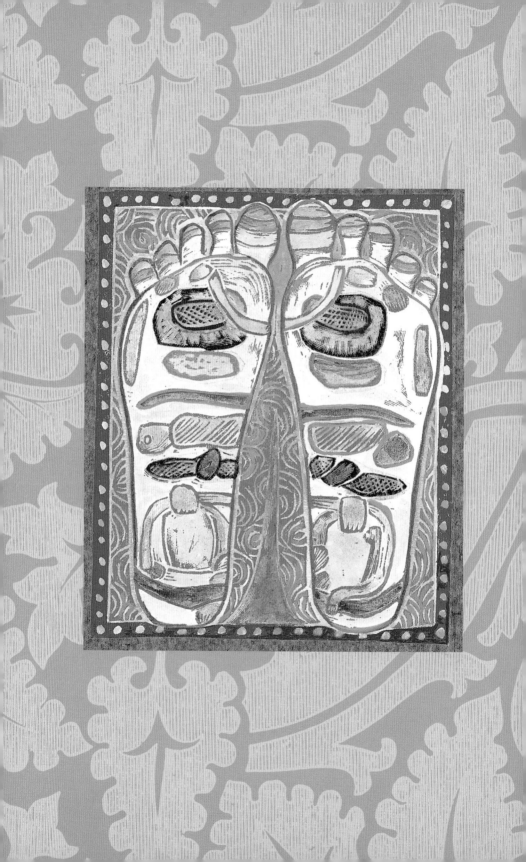

5

THE ZONES

Reflexology used to be called "zone therapy" because there are ten energy zones in the body, which run longitudinally from the base of the body (the feet) all the way to the top of the head.

This system is very much like the meridians in acupuncture, as the energy channels that run through the body are much the same as the zones. There are five zones on each side of the body.

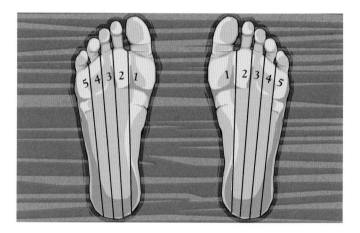

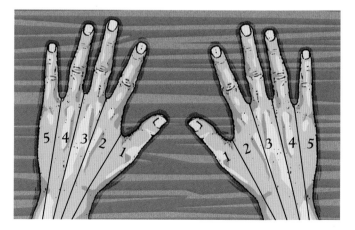

Energy lines and channels run through the body. Any blocked energy flow in the zones can affect the organs or systems that lie within that zone. This method of dividing the body into energy channels is thousands of years old and is the underlining principle of acupuncture. Along the meridians are acupuncture points that relate to different systems, and an impairment of energy flow through these zones or meridians will cause disease somewhere in the body. The blockages can cause stagnation and congestion that we can see in a variety of ways, from a painful joint to clogged sinuses.

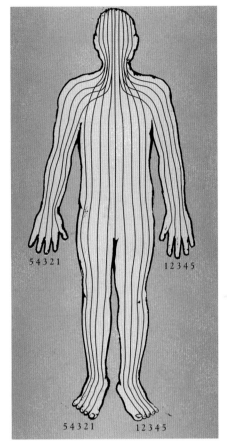

Though zones and meridians exist throughout the body, including in the hands and feet, reflexology concentrates on the body map that can be found on the feet, hands, and ears. Reflexology can disperse granular-type deposits in the meridian ends that are located in the hands and feet. After a while, you will no longer view feet as feet, because you will see the whole body mirrored on the feet. When I look at a foot, I see shoulders or a neck that is out of line, or pale areas in the digestive area, or puffiness in the bladder area.

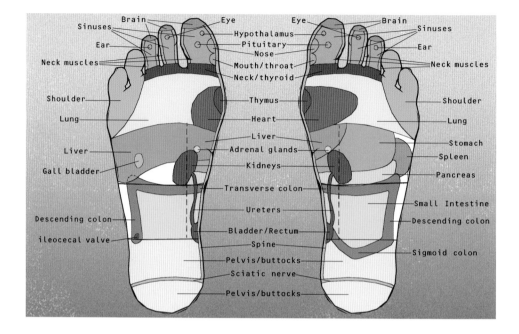

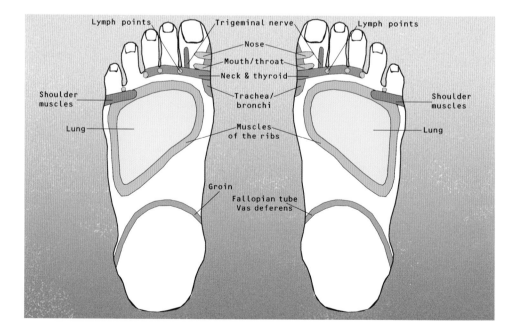

38

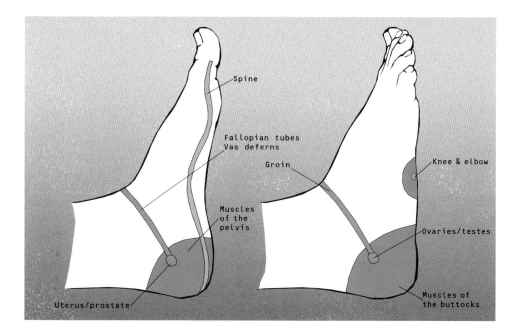

Spine

Fallopian tubes
Vas deferns

Groin

Knee & elbow

Muscles
of the
pelvis

Ovaries/testes

Uterus/prostate

Muscles of
the buttocks

YOUR FIRST STEP

At this point, I suggest that you find someone with whom you can practice reflexology. If that is absolutely impossible, set up a mirror so that you can see the soles of your own feet.

From a reflexology point of view, the soles of the feet are divided into three distinct areas. If it is possible, use a water-soluble felt-tipped pen or whiteboard marker and draw the lines on the feet so that you know exactly where the three areas are.

The area of the sole that reflexologists call the diaphragm line is commonly known as the balls of the feet. This area includes the toes, which relate to the head and neck areas, and the balls of the feet, which relate to the chest, heart, thymus, lung, and shoulder areas. The skin above the diaphragm line is generally darker than the skin below the line, so it is easy to see the dividing line. Don't be reluctant to draw the lines on your feet with a pen. I tell my students to do this, and they find it really helps. It is a good visual aid.

The waist line is found by locating the bone that protrudes a little on the outside of the foot. It is about halfway down the outside of the foot. Run your finger down the side of the foot until you feel a small protrusion. This protrusion is called the "metatarsal notch." Draw a line from this point straight across the bottom of the foot. The area from the diaphragm

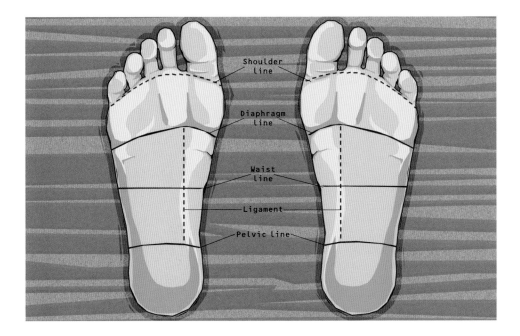

to the waist line relates to the liver, gall bladder, stomach, kidneys, adrenal glands, pancreas, and spleen.

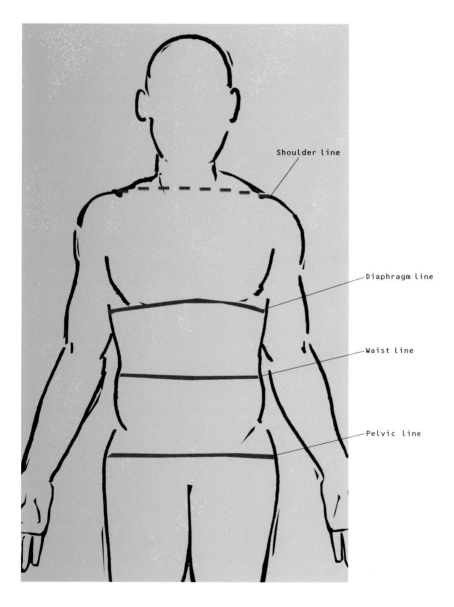

Shoulder line

Diaphragm line

Waist line

Pelvic line

The area that reflexologists call the pelvic line encompasses the area beneath the heel of the foot. If you look at the feet you will see how the color changes again from the middle area to the heel area, and this is where you will draw your line. Find the inside and the outside of the anklebone; the line is between these two points. The areas inside and outside the anklebone are reflex areas that relate to the bladder, small intestines, and large intestines. The heel area relates to the sciatic nerve and pelvic area.

If you look at the sole of the foot and pull all the toes up and back, you will see (or feel) the ligament that runs down the foot; it's like a tight cable. It is important when you first start to learn reflexology that you keep the foot relaxed, making sure you don't work over a tense ligament due to pulling the toes back, as this is not a pleasant experience.

HAND REFLEXOLOGY

As you will see in the next chapter, the hands can be treated like the feet, and there are some advantages to doing so. For example, it is easier to do reflexology on your own hands than on your own feet. You can treat a person's hands anywhere and at any time to help him or her with pain or to cope with a stressful situation, and you can give help to a work colleague during a difficult time. My husband and I work on each other's hands while on a long flight, as this helps our bodies to cope with jet lag.

Take care not to cause unnecessary problems, and never treat the hands if there is any broken skin, rashes, psoriasis, eczema, contact dermatitis, warts, or a fungal infection under the nails. When a palm reader touches a client's hands, he or she can avoid broken or damaged areas, but a reflexologist cannot, so don't touch hands or feet if you have any doubts at all.

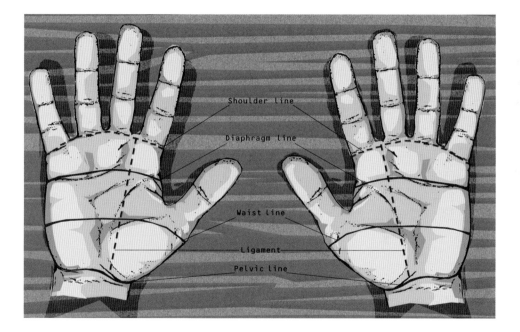

Shoulder line

Diaphragm line

Waist line

Ligament

Pelvic line

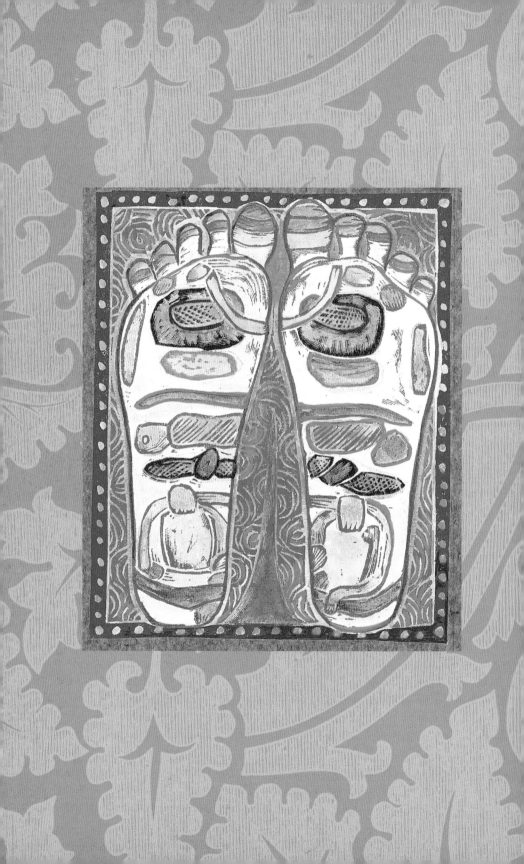

6

USING REFLEXOLOGY

FINGERNAILS

If you want to practice reflexology, long nails will be a thing of the past for you. I have had treatments that have been most unpleasant because the practitioner's nails have been in the way. This doesn't mean you have to cut your nails down to the quick. It does mean you have to be sensible; see what is comfortable for you and your guinea pig "patient," and you will soon discover the right working length. Even if your nails are short, it is still easy to dig into your client's skin with your nails if you use the top of your fingers or thumbs, so be careful how you place your fingers.

You need to learn to apply the correct movement to perform reflexology properly. A special technique is applied with the thumb or the index finger. Learning the technique needed for reflexology is very important, but it is also very simple, so it just takes practice. Though the movement is simple, it is very important to be thorough to cover the reflex points well, as there are thousands of them on both the hands and the feet.

The movement of the thumb or index finger is like a caterpillar moving forward. It is important to bear in mind that your finger or thumb should always be moving forward.

You need to use the ends of your fingers for this, but not the actual fingertips, as they are too harsh and the nails may accidentally dig into the client's foot. The movement is always forward and in tiny steps—about twelve tiny steps to an inch. Remember, the movement is steps, not sliding, and not circular. If you see the skin on your client's foot being pulled back while you are doing the caterpillar move, you are not moving forward; you must adjust and correct your movement.

How much pressure should you apply? That is a frequently asked question. At first, your fingers and thumbs will be weak and will tire easily, so there is no need to worry about applying too much pressure. Instead, concentrate on the technique. As your fingers and thumbs grow stronger and as you grow more confident, you will automatically start applying more pressure. As time goes on, this process will become intuitive, and you will know how much pressure feels good to the recipient. It is important that the pressure never become too strong, and that the person receiving the treatment isn't flinching. In reflexology or even massage there is what is known as "pleasant pain." What do we mean by "pleasant pain"? It's similar to a deep-tissue massage, where there is a certain amount of discomfort, but the very discomfort releases the muscles and makes the whole body feel so much better afterward. There are areas on a person's feet that may be tender, and reflexology will highlight this. The tenderness experienced is brief, however, as the thumb or finger passes over the area quickly.

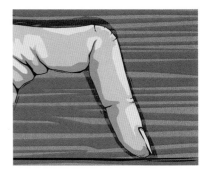

This position is too arched and is more likely to cause problems with nails digging in.

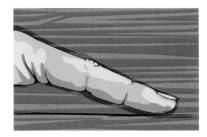

This position is too flat.

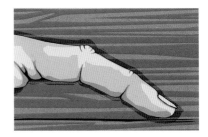

This position is correct.
Movement → Always forward
Never back
Never circular
Never sliding

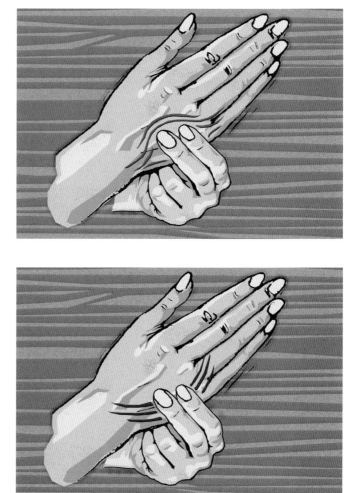

Correct

Incorrect

With experience you will get a feel for the feet. You need to be firm so as not to tickle the feet but not so firm as to turn someone off reflexology altogether. Just as we all like a different pressure from a massage, the same is true of a reflexology treatment. I like deep-tissue massage and I like deep reflexology, but I know plenty of people who prefer a lighter touch. Given time, this technique will become second nature, and you will gradually learn a smooth and consistent pressure.

Remember, the movement is always forward on the skin; if you see the skin just in front of the moving thumb or finger move backward, your technique is not correct. Remember to release the pressure slightly between each tiny caterpillar movement; this ensures the correct movement. Every time you have a minute, practice the movement on your own hands.

Tip:
1. Reflex points are tiny.
2. Movements should be tiny to cover all the reflex points.
3. The caterpillar movement is always forward, never backward.
4. Never use the top of your finger, as undoubtedly your nails will get in the way.
5. Never apply creams, oils, or lotions of any kind for the reflexology treatment. It is impossible to make good contact with the reflex points if the skin is at all slippery.
6. Remember to work slowly and methodically.
7. Practice makes perfect.

Practice this caterpillar walk on yourself at first, on your own hands. Sit down in a comfortable chair and put a cushion or pillow on your lap, as doing so will support your hands comfortably and at the right height for doing your work. To begin, practice for five minutes at a time, and you will begin to appreciate the way that the pressure and the technique feel. Eventually your fingers and thumbs will strengthen.

As you become more experienced, you will begin to feel changes in texture on the feet, such as a crunchy texture, deposits that feel like tiny crystals, air bubbles, or a popping sensation. These are areas of congestion, stagnation, or blocked energy. Sometimes the client feels soreness or pain. This pain or sensitivity is experienced only fleetingly, but it is an indication of an imbalance or blockage in the corresponding area of the body. It is not necessarily a major danger signal. For instance, a pain in the gall bladder reflex doesn't mean that this organ is about to stop functioning. In some cases it indicates scar tissue left when the gall bladder was surgically removed. It may simply mean the energy flow to that area needs balancing or that the patient is eating too many fatty, fried foods and putting his or her gall bladder under more strain than necessary.

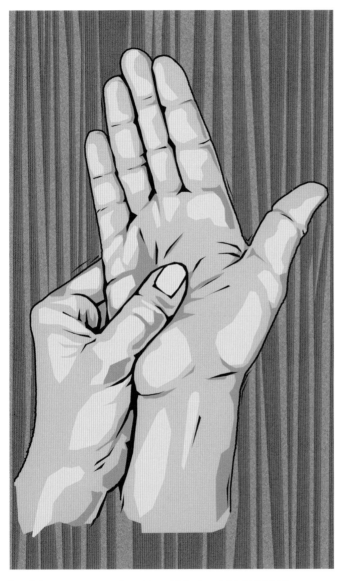

Feeling areas of congestion, stagnation, crystallization, or blocked energy in the hands.

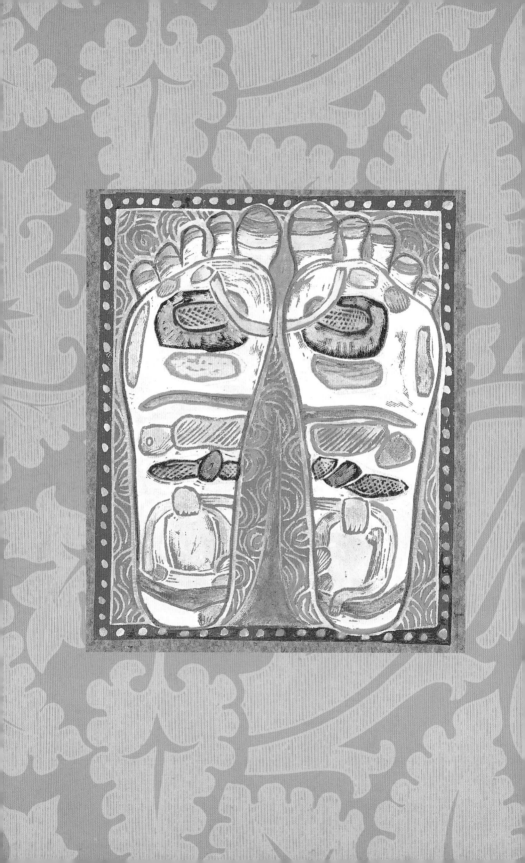

7

THE BALLS OF THE FEET

It is important to have a brief overview of how the body works. In recent years several teaching hospitals have taken reflexology on board by allowing reflexologists to give treatment to the patients on the wards. But we mustn't lose sight of the fact we are working on the physical, spiritual, and emotional levels and that we are more than the sum of our anatomical parts.

The foot area that runs from the bottom of the toes to the diaphragm line corresponds to the upper part of the trunk and all the organs that are located in that area. The shoulder blades and lower part of the shoulders are also included.

THE LUNGS

The lungs fill the chest area. They are light and spongy and they are involved in breathing. The left lung is slightly smaller than the right lung in order to accommodate the heart. In the lungs there is an exchange between oxygenated air and deoxygenated air. The lungs supply every cell with oxygen. Air is breathed in through the nose or mouth (preferably the nose) and warmed up and moistened as it passes through the nasal passage and pharynx, down through the trachea, or windpipe. The windpipe branches into two parts that are called "bronchi," and each bronchus takes air into one of the lungs. Inside the lung, the tube divides into many small tubes called the "bronchioles." At the end of these are pockets that resemble culs-de-sac, which are called "alveolar sacs." Under a microscope it is possible to see that each small alveolar sac is composed of tiny chambers called "alveoli." Their walls have a network of minute blood vessels called "capillaries," and it is here that there is an exchange of gases.

THE DIAPHRAGM

The diaphragm is a large sheet of muscle located at the bottom of the chest just below the lungs. It works with the intercostals, which are the muscles between the ribs. These are all designed to move the ribs in and out, squeezing and expanding the lungs and allowing us to breathe properly. The diaphragm and intercostals can become very tense and can hinder the movement necessary for breathing.

THE CHEST

The chest area consists of the ribs and the intercostals (the muscles between the ribs).

THE HEART

The heart pumps blood around the body to every cell. It beats more than one hundred thousand times a day! Make a fist; this is the approximate size of your heart. It is divided into two halves, with two chambers in each half and a valve that controls the blood flow between the two sides of the heart.

Deoxygenated blood enters the heart via the right atrium. It is then forced through the valve into the right ventricle. From there the blood is pumped to the lungs via the pulmonary artery. Oxygenated blood from the lungs travels back to the heart via the pulmonary veins, entering the left atrium, then the left ventricle, through the aorta, to be pumped around the body.

The heartbeat is controlled and managed by the autonomic nervous system. This is just as well, for it means we don't have to think about making the heart pump. While it's true that the heart pumps whether we think about it or not, we can influence it to a degree. Drinking caffeine or alcohol or drinking or eating anything containing saccharin can give us palpitations. Watching a horror movie can speed up the heartbeat, as does exercise. Chronic levels of stress hormones in the bloodstream will keep the heart beating faster than is ideal. Calm music, yoga, and breathing exercises can slow down the heartbeat. Reflexology can give the body the necessary impetus to encourage the heart to beat at the right pace. Each person is different and has his or her own unique set of imbalances.

THE CIRCULATION

The arteries are the largest of all the blood vessels in the body, and they transport oxygenated blood around the body. The smallest blood vessels are called "capillaries"; here blood passes through to the tissues to nourish the body, to remove waste fluids, and to remove deoxygenated blood.

After this, the capillaries flow into the veins and then back to the heart. If you want to know how fast your heart is beating, rest for a while and then take your pulse by counting the beats for one minute. Your heart should beat at approximately seventy beats per minute (a child's pulse is faster). A pulse between sixty and seventy beats per minute is better than one between seventy and eighty beats per minute.

Blood pressure is the pressure of blood exerted on the walls of the arteries. The perfect blood pressure is 120/80. Blood pressure can vary from day to day or from hour to hour. There are several reasons why a healthy person's blood pressure might go up. Exercise, stress, a heated argument, or what is known as "white coat syndrome" (when a patient's blood pressure goes up when a doctor or nurse takes it) may result in a temporary increase in blood pressure. If a nurse or doctor tells you that your blood pressure is high and that you should begin taking medication to lower it, it is worth buying a blood pressure monitor and checking your blood pressure several times a day under different circumstances at home over a period of several days. Some people find that their blood pressure varies a lot throughout the week or even during the course of a day. Reflexology can be a good treatment for low or high blood pressure.

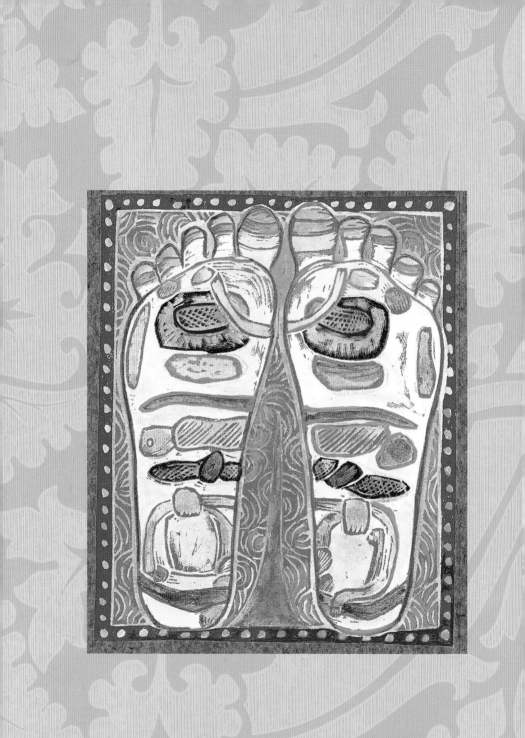

8

THE TOES

The toes correspond to the head, brain, ears, eyes, nose, sinuses, face, mouth, neck, and uppermost part of the shoulders. The big toe is the main area for the head. The big toe contains the reflex points for the pituitary gland, pineal gland, hypothalamus, brain, temples, upper and lower jaw, gums, teeth, throat, thyroid and parathyroid, and seven cervical vertebrae, which form the neck.

THE BRAIN

The brain is divided into several areas. The brain stem controls all our vital functions, such as breathing, blood pressure, and pulse rate. The cerebellum regulates sleep, consciousness, breathing, and circulation, and coordinates movement and balance. The brain is divided into right and left hemispheres. Together they control our intricate movements and communication skills. The left side of the cerebrum controls the right side of the body, as well as speech, language, writing, logic, mathematical skills, and analytical thinking. The right side of the cerebrum controls the left side of the body, as well as pattern perception, artistic ability, creativity, intuition, and nonverbal communication. It is important to exercise both the left and right hemispheres of the brain.

THE SINUSES

The sinuses are air-filled cavities in the head. They filter air that is breathed in through the mouth, and they help to lighten the weight of the head. The body has the lymphatic system for its drainage, whereas the head has the sinuses as its drainage system. Inflamed or even infected sinuses can cause anything from a stuffed-up feeling to severe head pain. Sinus problems can make breathing through the nose very difficult, if not impossible.

THE PITUITARY GLAND

The pituitary gland is like the conductor of an orchestra that plays a very complicated symphony. The gland, which is located behind the eyes and the nose, secretes hormones or controls the secretions of just about every hormone in the body. In other words, it has a direct or indirect affect on the whole endocrine system. The secretions from the pituitary gland affect growth, sexual development, fever, fainting, pregnancy and lactation, metabolism, mineral and sugar levels in the blood, fluid retention, energy levels, and much more.

THE PINEAL GLAND

The pineal gland is a small reddish-brown gland located in the front of the brain; it is connected to the brain by a stalk that contains nerves. This area responds to daylight and darkness and is responsible for releasing melatonin. The pineal gland plays a role in our moods and circadian rhythms (internal body clocks).

THE HYPOTHALAMUS

The hypothalamus regulates the autonomic nervous system; it controls emotions, reactions, appetite, and body temperature. The hypothalamus has the same reflex point as the pineal gland.

THE THYROID

The thyroid gland is located in the front of the neck; its hormones control our metabolism. The thyroid controls the rate at which the body uses nutrients, and it regulates calcium levels and protein building by the cells. Hypothyroidism, which means a low-functioning thyroid, causes the metabolism to slow down. A person with hypothyroidism puts on weight easily, and retains water. That person also moves, reacts, and thinks slowly. The face and body become bloated with excess fluids and the eyes become prominent. Hyperthyroidism refers to a thyroid that is functioning with the accelerator pedal pushed to the floor. Every function in the body is running fast. A person with this condition loses weight too easily.

THE PARATHYROIDS

The parathyroid glands are found at the thyroid location. They affect calcium and phosphorus levels, which are important for muscle function.

THE NECK

The neck contains seven cervical vertebrae, the lowest of which is usually somewhat prominent. With our lifestyles today, most people experience some sort of neck problem from time to time, sometimes chronic neck problems due to the muscles being tensed up all the time. This scenario can restrict the blood flow in the neck, reducing the amount of oxygen and nutrients that travels to the brain.

THE SHOULDERS

Only part of the shoulder area is located on this area of the feet. Due to our lifestyles these days, chronic aching shoulders are also a very common condition, like neck tension and tightness.

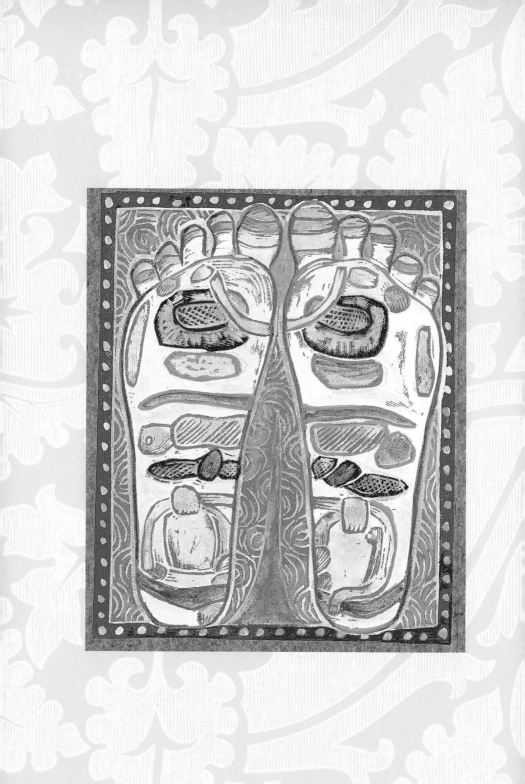

THE MIDDLE OF THE FOOT

The middle of the foot relates to the central part of the body and the organs in that area.

THE SOLAR PLEXUS

The solar plexus is a network of nerves located just in front of the stomach wall. This area is treated every time reflexology is performed, and treating this area creates a general feeling of well-being and a deep sense of relaxation. If you have ever experienced "butterflies in the stomach," you will know where the solar plexus is located. If a client is suffering emotional stress or if he or she is in constant pain, this area will be tender. Pain is extremely draining and can cause a lot of physical and emotional stress. Chronic pain disturbs sleep patterns, which in turn causes more stress and hence more pain. It's a vicious circle. Reflexology can help redress this problem and break the circle.

THE DIGESTIVE SYSTEM

It was well-known to the ancients that a good working digestive system is the foundation to good health and a long life, and this is still true. You may eat a nutritious diet, but if your digestion and ability to absorb nutrients are impaired, it will totally undermine everything you are trying to achieve. The body has many ways of telling you the digestive system is struggling. Determine whether the following symptoms are happening more than just occasionally:

- Bloating
- Burping
- Gas
- Reflux (heartburn)
- Discomfort
- Pain
- Constipation
- Diarrhea

Reflexology is a very effective way of balancing a distressed digestive system. These days, digestive problems are common because we eat nutrient-deficient foods and foods that are hard to digest. We consume too many stimulants and often eat on the run and under stress. Our digestive systems need a helping hand (literally), and reflexology can treat every organ, system, and tissue to support better digestive function.

THE LIVER

The liver is the largest organ in the body and has to perform hundreds of functions. An adult liver weighs about four pounds. It is located on the right side of the upper abdomen, where it is protected by the ribs. The liver has about five hundred different functions that range from producing bile and cholesterol to breaking down many toxic substances, such as pharmaceutical medications or alcohol, and converting them into less harmful substances so the body can dispose of them more efficiently. The liver is a major detoxifying organ. It processes nutrients from the blood, and it stores fats, sugars, and proteins until the body needs them. The gall bladder is a small organ that stores the bile that the liver has produced. Bile is released into the small intestines, where it helps break down fat and fat-soluble vitamins, enabling us to absorb these vital nutrients.

THE STOMACH

The stomach is located a little to the left side of the body under the rib cage. It breaks down food and begins protein digestion by releasing gastric juices.

THE PANCREAS

The pancreas sits behind the stomach, mostly on the left side of the body, and is about six inches long. There are two parts to this organ. One part helps to control blood sugar levels by producing the hormone insulin, which most people have heard of and associate with diabetes. The other part of the pancreas produces digestive enzymes: Lipase breaks down fats, protease breaks down proteins, and amylase breaks down carbohydrates. The pancreas sends these enzymes into the small intestine, where digestion continues after food has left the stomach.

THE SPLEEN

The spleen is located on the left side of the body under the diaphragm and behind the stomach. Part of the lymphatic system, it produces lymphocytes and filters out damaged or worn-out red blood cells. It filters the lymph, removing toxins and bacteria, and produces antibodies. This organ is a very important part of our immune system. The spleen area can be found two finger widths above the "waist line" on the left foot.

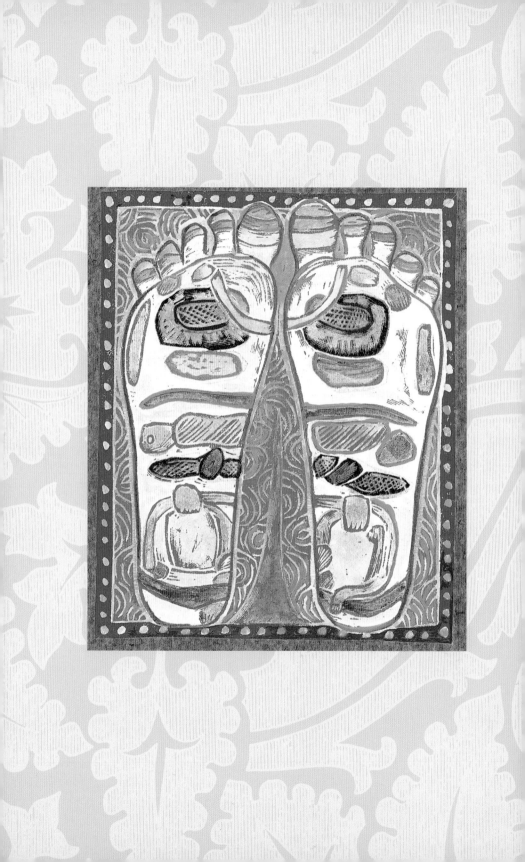

10

THE WAIST LINE

The waist line area is below the notch on the side of the foot.

THE SMALL INTESTINE

Now we move to the part of the sole that is still under the instep but that starts to creep under the heel area. This part of the sole relates to the lower digestive system, starting with the small intestine. The small intestine is like a long pipe or tube approximately twenty-two feet long. It is like a food-processing conveyor belt. The first part of the small intestine, the duodenum, is about twelve inches long. The duodenum receives the digestive enzymes made by the pancreas. The stomach empties its contents into the duodenum, and these contents must be neutralized immediately; otherwise, the acidic nature of the stomach contents will burn the lining of the duodenum, causing duodenal ulcers. The next section of the small intestine, the jejunum, is about eight feet long, and the last section, the ileum, is about twelve feet long. It is here in the small intestine that most nutrients are absorbed.

THE ILEOCECAL VALVE

The ileocecal valve lies between the small and large intestines; it prevents fecal matter from backing up into the small intestine.

THE APPENDIX

The appendix is located at the beginning of the large intestine. It helps to lubricate the colon and is thought to secrete antibodies. The appendix is not vital to our health, so once it causes a problem, it is vital to have it removed.

THE LARGE INTESTINE (COLON)

The large intestine is actually shorter than the small intestine; it is only five feet in length, but it is called the "large intestine" because it is a wider tube than the small intestine. This U-shaped tube is divided into the ascending colon, the transverse colon, the descending colon, and the sigmoid colon. It absorbs water and removes mucus and waste matter. Constipation is a common problem, and in many cases there is an emotional component to this problem, especially with women. Our modern diet and lifestyle don't help.

The Sigmoid Colon
The sigmoid colon is the last part of the large intestine before waste enters the rectum.

THE URINARY AREA

The urinary system consists of the bladder, urethras, and kidneys.

The Kidneys

The kidneys are located at the back of the body on either side of the spine, above the waist and under the rib cage for protection. They are our main filtering organs. They filter toxins and waste products from the blood, and they produce urine for excretion via the bladder. They also regulate the balance of fluids and minerals in the body. Blood enters the kidneys through the medulla from the renal artery. Once filtered, the fluid passes to the tubules, which are surrounded by capillaries. The tiny capillaries remove most the water and useful chemicals and minerals that will go back into the bloodstream via the renal vein. The waste that is left behind is then passed from the kidneys to the urinary bladder via the urethra. Your kidneys can process around forty-two gallons of blood a day!

The Bladder

The bladder is a hollow muscular bag located just behind the hip bone. At the bottom of the bladder is the urethral sphincter; this structure keeps the fluid in the bladder until it is full and the bladder is ready to empty. Urine leaves the bladder via a tube called the "urethra." We get signals to empty our bladders once there is about a cup full, but the bladder can hold up to a pint of fluid, if necessary.

ADRENAL GLANDS

There are two adrenal glands; these small glands, which are involved in more than fifty different functions, sit on top of the kidneys. The adrenal glands produce hormones involved in stress, increased heart rate, vasoconstriction, increased breathing rate, and increased muscle contraction. The adrenal glands also produce hormones that have an anti-inflammatory effect on the whole body. They are involved in sexual development, allergies, and energy. These glands also help to support the system after menopause. Our lifestyles put these overworked and underrated glands under enormous amounts of stress.

THE SPINE

The backbone is extremely complex; it affects every function in the body. It is made up of vertebrae, which are small bones that fit together to protect the spinal cord but leave it mobile enough so we have flexibility. There are seven cervical vertebrae that form the neck, twelve thoracic vertebrae that form the back, and five lumber vertebrae that form the lower back, plus the sacrum and coccyx, which are made up of vertebrae fused together at the bottom of the spine.

The spinal cord is housed in this spinal column for its protection. It feeds the entire body with nerves, constantly sending messages to and receiving messages from the brain, subconsciously and consciously controlling and coordinating all the functions of the entire body. So any problems in the spine could cause a problem in the relevant part of the body, organ, or system relating to the area in the spine that is affected. Pay special attention to the spine, and make sure you work this reflex zone thoroughly, as this will affect every cell in the body for the better.

Aches and pains in and around the spine are common. We generally have poor posture, we spend too much time over a computer or slouching in front of the television, and we pick up heavy items incorrectly. Most people are dehydrated, leaving muscles stiff and pulling the spine out of alignment. It is common to see people with neck ache, middle backache, or lower backache. A problem in the spine or the muscles surrounding the spine could contribute to a condition or could be the cause of the condition.

SCIATIC NERVE

The sciatic nerve is not a reflex point on the foot but the extremity of the actual sciatic nerve. The sciatic nerve runs from the buttocks down the leg to the base of the heel. The sciatic nerve can become inflamed when the contents of a torn disk press on it or when fluid surrounding a torn muscle presses on it; this causes pain to run down the leg. This complaint is a common one that we often enounter at our clinic.

DERMATOMES AND MYOTOMES

The spine also relates to dermatomes, which are areas on the skin. Myotomes are areas that relate to muscles.

Every part of our skin is supplied with sensory neurons that carry messages from the skin to the spinal cord and finally to the brain. When some part of the skin is stimulated but the sensation is not felt, the nerves supplying that dermatome are most likely damaged or inflamed, which provides us with information regarding which part of the spinal cord could be damaged or inflamed. The myotomes are similar to dermatomes. If the area is paralyzed, or partially paralyzed, the motor neurons in that spinal section may well be damaged or inflamed.

If you come across a client whose hands and feet have numb areas, it would be a good idea to refer that person to a qualified registered osteopath or chiropractor for further investigation.

THE FEMALE REPRODUCTIVE SYSTEM

The female reproductive system consists of a uterus, two fallopian tubes, and two ovaries.

The Ovaries

Healthy ovaries produce a ripe egg once a month. An egg leaves the ovary via the fallopian tube and enters the uterus. The ovaries also produce estrogen, which begins to diminish with age. By the time women reach the late forties and early fifties, the ovaries will have stopped producing estrogen, although the body does still produce small amounts from fat cells and the adrenal glands.

The Fallopian Tubes

The fallopian tubes propel the egg to the uterus by the movement of tiny threadlike protrusions that have peristaltic-type muscular contractions (a wavelike movement).

The Uterus

The uterus is situated at the top of the vagina, behind the urinary bladder. The uterus is held in place by a series of muscles and ligaments attached to the pelvic floor and the pelvis. The function of this organ is to incubate a baby, so a thickly interwoven wall of muscle fibers protects it.

THE MALE REPRODUCTIVE SYSTEM

The male reproductive organs consist of two testes, the prostate gland, and the vas deferens (the tube through which semen and sperm pass).

The Prostate Gland

The prostate gland is located at the first part of the urethra at the base of the bladder. Its secretions give the sperm something to swim in. This organ can become swollen or inflamed, which is a common problem as men get older, causing the need for frequent urination.

The Testes

The testes are two organs that are located outside the body so they stay cool. The testes produce about fifty million sperm a day. The seminal vesicle stores the mature sperm. These glands also produce testosterone, the hormone that gives men their male characteristics.

MUCOUS MEMBRANES

The mucous membranes are found in the reproductive system, digestive system, and respiratory system. There is a reflex connection that links the different mucous membranes, so generally speaking, if one is affected, they can all be affected.

Mucus is produced to protect the body from the outside from foreign invaders. This may be a strange comment for you to appreciate at first, but the mucous membranes are the "outside" of your body! When molecules have passed into the bloodstream, we can refer to the "inside" of the body. So the air we breathe in passes to the lungs, where the mucous lining catches particles such as pollen and dust. The food we ingest is definitely perceived by the body as foreign until it is broken down into recognizable molecules. If we keep eating foods that are unhealthy, the mucous lining will produce more mucus to protect itself. This could have a detrimental affect on overall digestion and absorption of nutrients.

THE LYMPHATIC SYSTEM

The lymphatic system is found throughout the body and is closely interconnected with the circulatory system. You automatically treat the lymphatic system when you are working on other reflex points on the feet. The lymphatic system is part of our immune system, and it consists of a network of vessels that are distributed throughout the body.

From time to time we may experience swellings in the neck, armpit, or groin. You may have even described these as "swollen glands," but they are actually inflamed lymph nodes. They swell when the body's white blood cells gather en masse to fight, destroy, and absorb harmful substances such as bacteria.

SKELETAL AREA

Reflex zones for the skeletal system are found in many areas on the feet. The many bones in the body give structure to the body, protect organs, and, with help of muscles, enable us to move. The bones are classified into long bones, short bones, flat bones, and irregularly shaped bones. Bones are not solid; they have a hard exterior and a spongy interior, which makes them strong but light. Bones are composed mainly of calcium and phosphorus, but they also contain many other nutrients and minerals. Bones also act as a store of calcium for the bloodstream. When our systems become too acidic, the body releases calcium reserves in the bones to help neutralize this acidity in the blood and elsewhere in the body.

THE MUSCULAR AREA

Reflex zones for the muscular system are found in many areas of the feet. As you work the feet, you will automatically be working the muscles. They come in three types: the skeletal muscles, which we can move and which are also called the "voluntary muscles"; the smooth muscles, which are known as involuntary muscle, and which ensure that our organs are working automatically even when we are asleep; and the cardiac muscle, which also works automatically.

THE NERVOUS SYSTEM

The spine, brain, and solar plexus form the major parts of the nervous system. The whole nervous system is treated every time reflexology is performed. The central nervous system includes the brain and the spinal cord. The peripheral nervous system includes the autonomic nervous system. The solar plexus reflex point helps to calm and relax the whole nervous system.

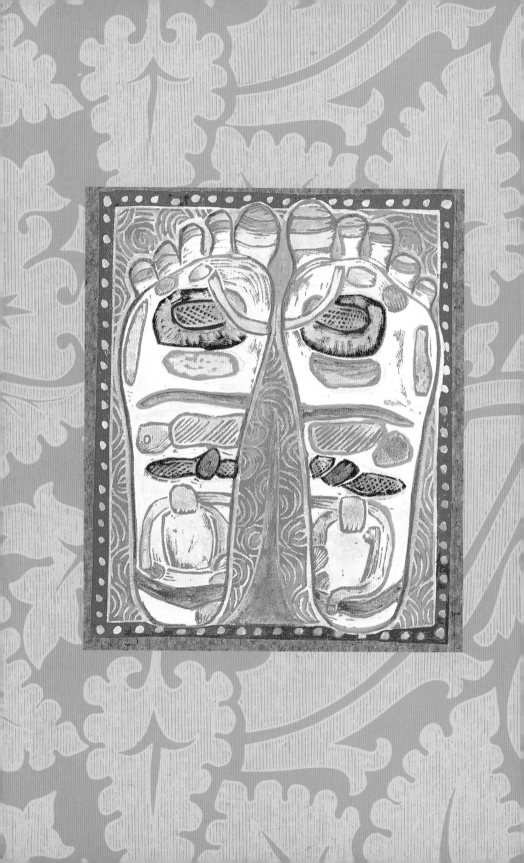

11

GETTING STARTED

EQUIPMENT THAT YOU WILL NEED

You will need the following things for your reflexology work. Some of these items are essential, but large and expensive things, such as treatment couches, are not necessary at this stage.

Powder

Powder is important in reflexology treatments; however, talcum powder can damage the lungs when inhaled, so use corn flour or arrowroot powder, for example. Reflexology is performed on feet or hands that have been lightly dusted with powder. This enables you to have a good grip and better control, as it is impossible to do the technique correctly if the feet are covered in oil, as you will lose contact. If you would like to add something extra to your treatment, after the reflexology portion is complete, you may use a little coconut oil or almond oil with some added essential oils to massage the feet for a few minutes. (See Chapter 13, "Self-Help and Essential Oils," for information on essential oils and how to enhance a treatment or create a healing atmosphere.)

Towels

Have handy some towels or sheets to keep the feet warm and surfaces clean. Keep some washable thin cotton blankets or some very large towels available for those people who feel the cold more than others. Relaxing for an hour can make some people feel cooler than usual.

Treatment Tables

A good treatment table makes the treatment more comfortable for the recipient and makes it much easier for you to perform the reflexology treatment. (You don't want to end up with back problems yourself while helping others.) If you do decide to buy a table, make sure it is adjustable. However, a treatment table is not imperative if funds are in short supply. As a matter of interest, I decided to go on the Internet recently and typed in "secondhand treatment table"; I found many at very reasonable prices. For instance, I saw an adjustable table in very good condition for one hundred dollars. Generally, static tables are cheaper than portable (fold-up for carrying or storing) tables. If you buy a static table, you will need somewhere to keep it. Remember, even if the vinyl on the table is not in good condition, the table is always covered in sheets and towels; metal legs can be painted, and wooden legs can be rubbed down and varnished. I bought my static adjustable reflexology table secondhand many years ago for fifty dollars, and I still use it. All I had to do was paint the metal legs. If you have a choice, buy an adjustable table.

Other Items

In addition to a comfortable table, the following help to make the reflexology experience soothing and pleasant.

- Three or four pillows
- A stool or an office chair on wheels, which can also be bought secondhand
- Music—anything from classical to instrumental to New Age

- An aromatherapy burner to warm up essential oils to create a healing atmosphere
- Disposable cups, because you should provide your client with a glass of water after the treatment
- Tissues, because sometimes treatment can make people's noses run (this could be due to the sinuses being encouraged to clear), and sometimes treatment can release or unblock emotions that make people cry (this is not common)

If a lack of money or space makes a special table impossible, try the following:

It you have a strong kitchen table, use that. Get a piece of foam cut to size (it can be rolled away afterward)—this will make it quite comfortable—or use a thick quilt, plus plenty of pillows. It is important to place a pillow under the client's knees to take the stress off the back. You sit on an office chair or stool on wheels.

You could use your sofa. Have your client lie down and put his or her feet over the end of the armrest; this will raise the feet high enough for you to treat them comfortably—certainly higher than a bed. Use plenty of pillows, including one under the knees. You sit on a low stool.

You could use a bed, again placing a pillow under your client's knees; however, treatment can be difficult as beds can be too low for you to perform the treatment comfortably (remember your back).

My least favorite option is to put your client in an armchair with you sitting in another chair opposite your client. Place your client's feet on your lap. This position can place a strain on his or her knees and back, however, as they are not supported properly. This position could also become very uncomfortable for you, as you will not be able to move around, which could give you back problems. Overall, I do not recommend this setup.

STARTING POINT FOR GIVING TREATMENTS

For the sake of simplicity, I refer here to the person you work on as your "client," but you might want to think of that person as your patient or even a relative or friend. Again, for the sake of simplicity, in this chapter I assume that your client is female.

After you have welcomed your client, ask her to take off her shoes and socks. Help her to settle down comfortably with enough pillows behind her back and knees to take the strain off her back and hips. I mention this a few times because it is important to take any strain off the body while you are treating someone. Ask your client whether she would prefer to be covered with a large towel or a cotton blanket.

Take a look at your client's feet. Can you see any cuts, blisters, rashes, fungal infections, or open sores? If you do see these things, you may have to abandon the idea of treating the feet for the time being and work on the hands instead. To be honest, most people don't come for treatment with their feet in such a condition. If they have practical problems of this kind, they usually wait until their feet have healed.

Now is a good time to ask some questions. Ask your client whether she is pregnant, has a pacemaker, or is diabetic. It is best not to treat pregnant or diabetic clients until you are extremely well trained and experienced.

Then cover both feet lightly with a powder of your choice (but not talcum powder). It is important to remember that while you are treating one foot, you should always leave the other foot covered with a towel. Occasionally a client will ask to have her foot left uncovered if she is feeling hot or if she is having a hot flash.

For beginners, it is very helpful to draw the lines on the feet, as described previously. Within no time you will see these invisible sections on the feet without drawing the lines.

Then settle down and focus your attention on the treatment; clear your mind.

Always begin with some relaxation techniques.

RELAXATION TECHNIQUES

The first two relaxation methods are the only ones that you perform while standing.

- Gently but firmly put your hands under and around the back of the patient's heels, cradling the heels in the palms of your hands. Lean back a little, raise the legs off the table just a fraction, and slowly stretch the legs. Leaning back will allow the weight of your body to do the work of stretching. This slow, gentle movement helps to release tension in the lower back and hips. Repeat this a few times.
- Maintaining your hold but not the stretching, and this time keeping the client's legs on the table, rock both feet from side to side, both in the same direction, just like windshield wipers. Do this about four or five times. This relaxes the client's lower back.

Following are a variety of relaxation techniques you could use at the start of, during, or at the end of your reflexology treatment. There are also many you will discover for yourself. Experiment, finding your own unique movements; you can enlist the help of a friend to tell you what feels good. The rest of the reflexology treatments described here are always preformed sitting down; only the leg stretch and lower-back relaxation are performed standing.

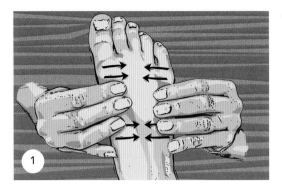

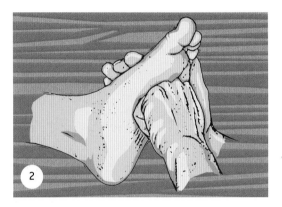

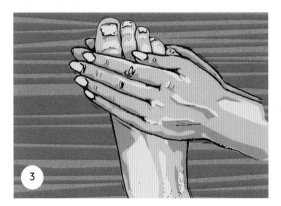

- **Technique 1:** Place both your thumbs under the foot, and then place all your fingers on top of the foot. Starting at the base of the foot, move all your fingers using the caterpillar walk technique across the top of the foot. Allow your fingers to come close to each other but not to meet, or you might pinch the client's skin. Repeat this process, moving up the foot. Most people love this technique. Return to the beginning and repeat two or three times more.

- **Technique 2:** Place your right hand on top of the left foot; make a fist with your left hand and place it on the ball of the foot. Alternately push with your fist and squeeze with your hand. Repeat this a few times.

- **Technique 3:** Using both hands, sandwich the foot. Rotate both hands, gently squeezing them together. Repeat this two or three times more.

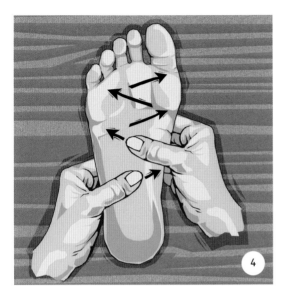

- **Technique 4:** Pass your thumbs, alternating left and right, over the client's foot in long sweeping movements, moving up and down the length of the foot. Repeat a few times.

- **Technique 5:** Move your thumbs together straight across the client's foot—moving up or down the foot. Repeat this a few times.

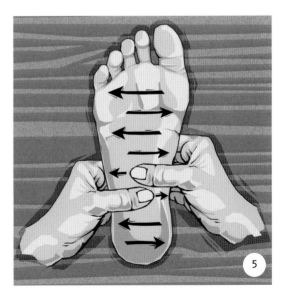

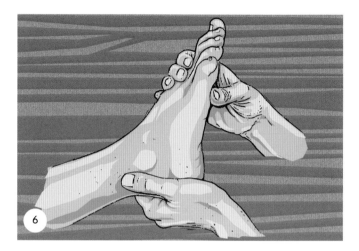

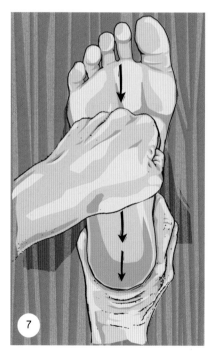

- **Technique 6:** Place your left hand under the client's right heel, with your right hand over the foot and your thumb under the right foot (thumb facing straight toward the little toe). Gently rotate the foot at the ankle in both directions a few times.

- **Technique 7:** Make a fist and move down the foot in a long sweeping movement. Repeat this a few times.

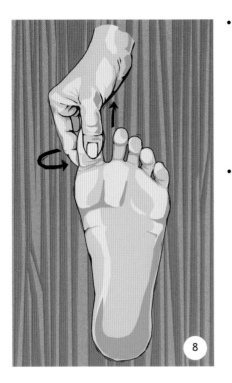

- **Technique 8:**
  Gently stretch one toe at a time; then rotate it to loosen the joint.

- **Technique 9:**
  Place your palms one either side of the foot. Alternately slide your hands up and down the sides of the feet. Repeat a few times.

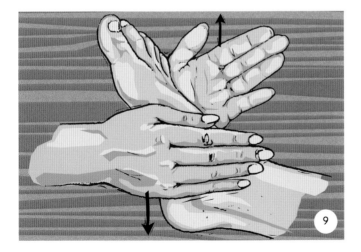

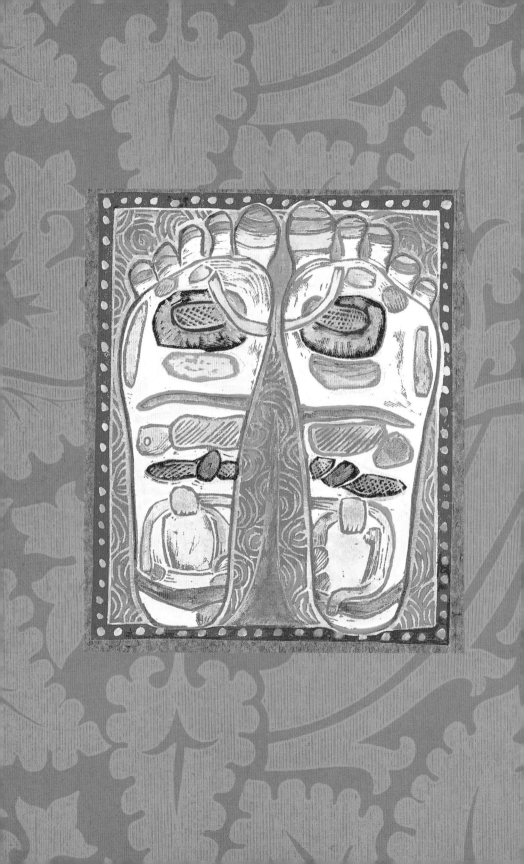

12

FOOT REFLEXOLOGY

TREATING THE REFLEXES OF THE LUNGS, CHEST, HEART, AND SHOULDERS

Take the right foot in your left hand and put your thumb on the upper part of the diaphragm area. Then use the thumb of your right hand to move upward to the toes in a caterpiller movement. Now change hands and do the same thing again.

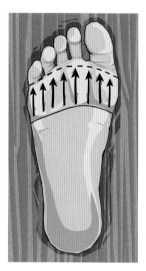

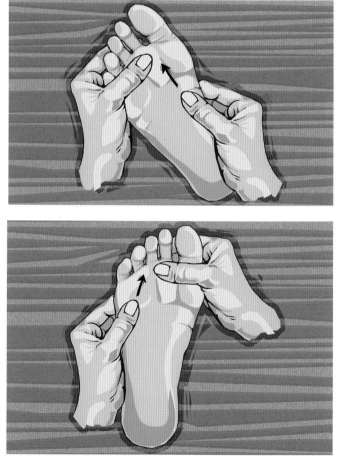

RELAXATION TECHNIQUE

Add a relaxation technique at this point. Choose any one of the relaxation techniques described earlier, or use one of your own, before moving on to the next stage. A relaxation technique is a handy thing to do if you forget where you are in the treatment, which can easily happen if the client asks questions during treatments.

TREATING THE REFLEXES OF THE SINUSES, NECK, PART OF THE HEAD, AND SHOULDERS

The next area to be treated is the toe area. This is a little more involved.

Holding the right foot with your left hand, use your right thumb to caterpillar walk up the large toe; you will need to walk up the large toe about four or five times, working from the base to the top to cover the whole area. Using the right index finger, work up the side of the next toe; then use the thumb to work up the middle of that toe. Use the right index finger to work up the side of the next toe, and then use your thumb to walk up the middle of that toe. Keep repeating this process until you reach the little toe. Change hands and work up the middle of the toe with the left thumb, change to the left index finger and work up the side of the toe, and repeat until you reach the end of the large toe.

It sounds complicated, but it isn't really. Remember this system:

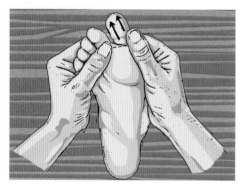

1. Right thumb up the middle of the toe
2. Right index finger up the right side of the toe
3. On the return, left thumb up the middle of the toe
4. Left index finger up the left side of the toe

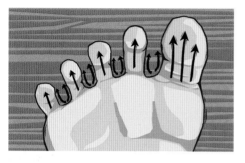

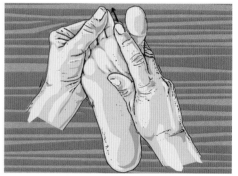

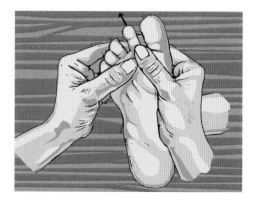

TREATING THE REFLEXES OF THE EYES AND EARS

Hold the right foot with your left hand; then, with your right thumb and fingers, pull up the toe that is next to the large toe. Now gently but firmly rotate the thumb in the fleshy part of the toe three times. Do the same with the next toe.

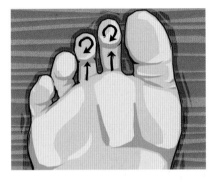

Note: You can use a rotating movement when working on the toes, but not on other parts of the foot.

TREATING THE REFLEXES OF THE NECK AND THYROID

Hold the right foot in your left hand and work with the right thumb across the base of the first three toes. Starting the caterpillar walk from the base of the big toe to the base of the third toe, repeat this movement twice more.

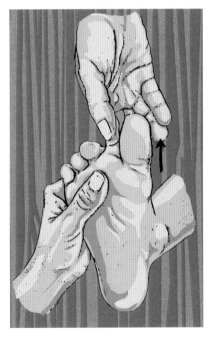

Now make a fist with your left hand and place it on the balls of the feet as shown on the diagram on the next page. With your right index finger and second finger, work across the base of the first three toes on the front of the right foot, starting with the big toe. Repeat this twice more.

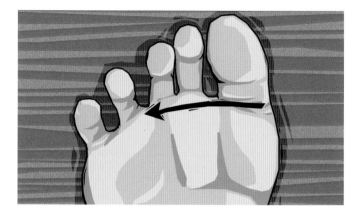

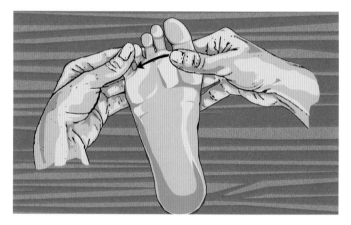

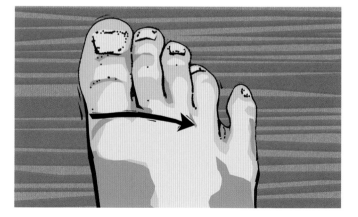

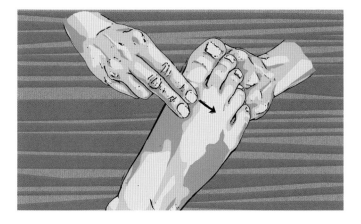

TREATING THE REFLEXES OF THE FACE

Maintain the position of your left fist supporting the right foot under the ball of the foot, and using only the index finger of your right hand, work across the large toe. Stop before you reach the nail bed of the big toe. Repeat this twice more.

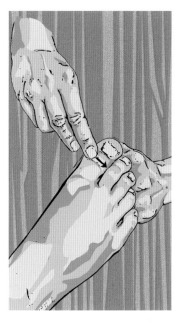

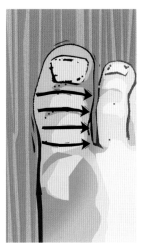

TREATING THE REFLEXES OF THE CHEST

Hold the client's foot in one hand, then use the index finger of the other hand to caterpiller walk downward from the toes and across the diaphragm area.

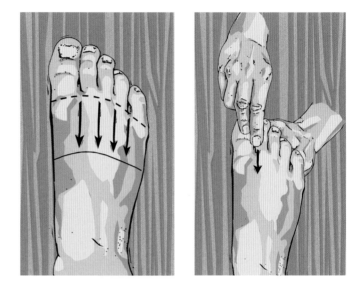

RELAXATION TECHNIQUE

Use another relaxation technique at this point; choose one different from the first.

TREATING THE REFLEXES OF THE LIVER AND GALL BLADDER

Ninety percent of the liver's reflex area is found on the right foot. Hold the right foot in your left hand and work the area from the diaphragm line to the waist line, at the angle shown in the diagram.

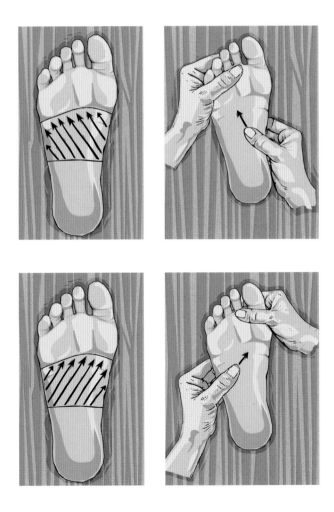

TREATING THE REFLEXES OF THE STOMACH, PANCREAS, AND SPLEEN

Hold the left foot in your right hand and work the area from the diaphragm line to the waist line. Cradle the heel from below.

RELAXATION TECHNIQUE

Use another relaxation technique now; choose one different from the first two.

TREATING THE REFLEXES OF THE ILEOCECAL VALVE, SMALL INTESTINE, AND LARGE INTESTINE

On the right foot, find the reflex for the ileocecal valve by the pelvic line on the outside edge of the foot. Cradling the heel in your right hand, apply pressure with your left thumb. While still applying pressure, pull the thumb back toward the outside edge. Do this three times. Change hands when yours become tired.

Now work the area from the waist line down, using your right thumb to work across the area in the direction indicated on the diagram on the next page. Work across until you get to the end of the foot. Change hands, so that now you cradle the right foot in your right hand and use your left thumb to work across the area down to the end.

TREATING THE REFLEX OF THE SIGMOID COLON

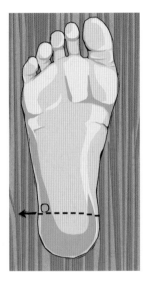

Cradle the left heel in your right hand. Using your thumb, start at the center of the sole under the instep and rub your thumb firmly across the foot to the outside edge of the sole.

Now work the area from the waist line down, using your left thumb to work across the area in the direction indicated on the diagram. Work across until you get to the end of the foot. Change hands, and use your right thumb to work across the area down to the end.

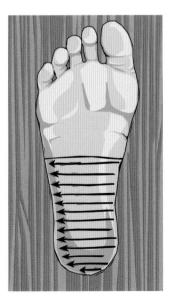

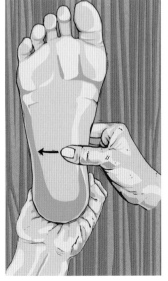

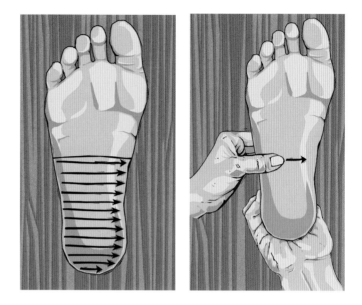

RELAXATION TECHNIQUE

Use another relaxation technique at this point; choose one different from the first three.

TREATING THE REFLEXES OF THE SPINE AND THE HIP AND PELVIS AREA

Support the right foot with the left hand approximately halfway down the outside edge. With your right thumb work up the inside of the foot, following the arch contour. As you work up the inside with your right thumb you will need to bring your fingers around to the front of the foot. Work from

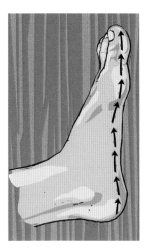

the bottom of the foot all the way up to finish at the top, along the side of the big toe. Start from the beginning and repeat two more times.

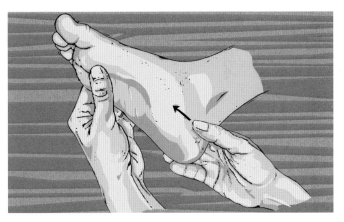

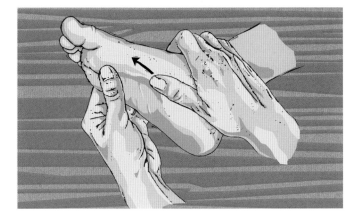

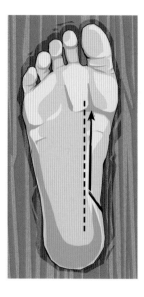

TREATING THE REFLEXES OF THE KIDNEY, BLADDER, AND ADRENAL GLANDS

If you look along the reflex of the spine just as the arch begins, you will see a slightly puffy area (in some people it is very puffy); this is the bladder reflex point. Holding the right foot with your left hand, use your right thumb and, starting at the bladder point, move toward the ligament line and work up this side of the ligament line, but not on the ligament itself. Be mindful to keep the ligament relaxed; otherwise, you will cause your client discomfort. Stop when you reach the adrenal gland area, which is approximately under the second finger width from the diaphragm. Return your thumb to the bladder reflex point, repeat this twice more, and finally rotate the adrenal reflex point three times.

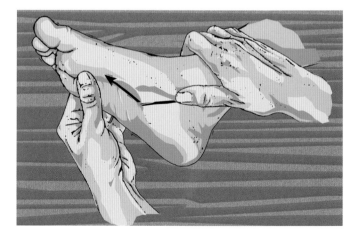

TREATING THE REFLEXES OF THE REPRODUCTIVE SYSTEM

Holding the right foot in your right hand, work with your left thumb from the tip of the heel on the outside of the foot to the anklebone. Repeat this twice more. Change hands, holding the right foot with your left hand, and work your right thumb from the tip of the heel on the inside of the foot to the anklebone. Repeat this twice more.

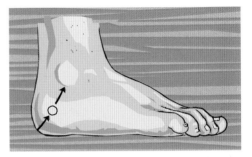

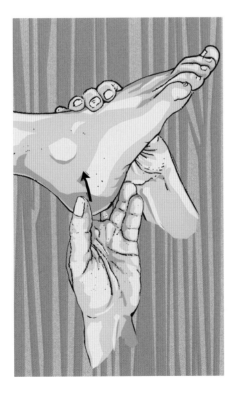

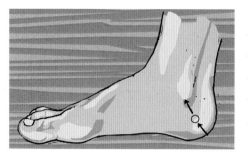

Support the right foot by placing both thumbs on the sole of the foot; then, with the first two fingers of each hand, work on top of the foot. Start at each anklebone and work around the ankle until your fingers almost meet in the middle. Repeat this two more times.

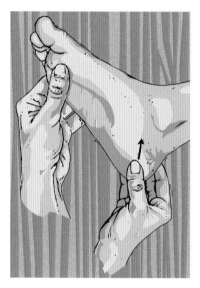

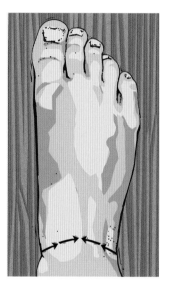

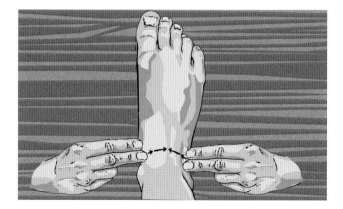

TREATING THE REFLEXES OF THE COCCYX

Cradle and wrap the heel of the right foot with your left hand, and support the upper part of the foot with your right hand. Use your four fingers as shown in the diagram to work across the inside of the heel.

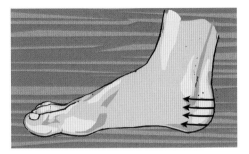

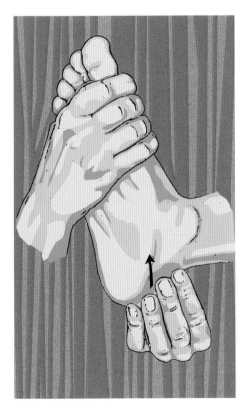

TREATING THE REFLEXES OF THE HIPS AND PELVIS

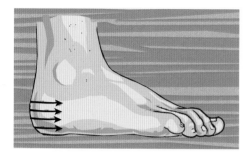

Change hands so that you take the right foot in your right hand, cradling and wrapping the heel. Support the upper part of the foot with your left hand, and use your four fingers to work across the outside of the heel.

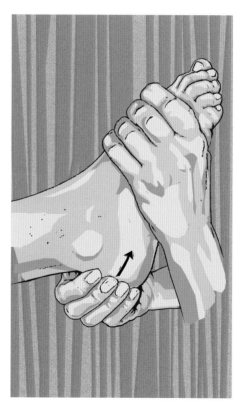

TREATING THE REFLEXES OF THE SHOULDER

Support the right foot with your right fist. Use your left index finger to work across from the outside across two toe widths, continue down to the diaphragm line as indicated in the diagram, and repeat two more times.

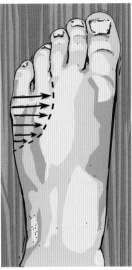

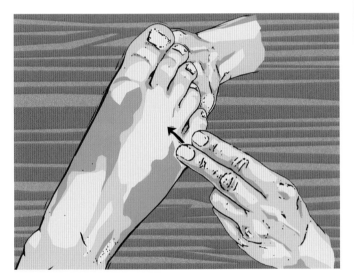

TREATING THE REFLEXES OF THE ARM, KNEE, AND ELBOW

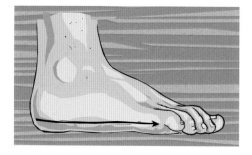

Support the right foot with your right hand, using your left thumb to work up the outside of the foot from the heel to the base of the little toe. Repeat this once more.

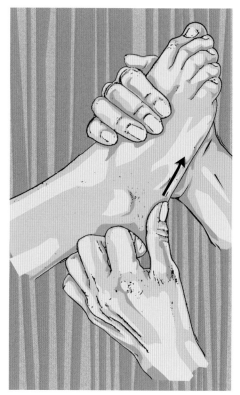

FINISHING THE TREATMENT ON THE RIGHT FOOT

Finish the treatment with some relaxation techniques. Cover the right foot with a towel.

AT THE END OF THE REFLEXOLOGY TREATMENT

Finally, on the left foot, finish with a relaxation technique. At this point you could use massage oil or lotion with essential oils to do a brief foot massage on both feet. For this you would use smooth, gliding movements. Gently wipe off the excess oil with a towel when you have finished. The oil and massage are an optional part of the treatment.

Give the recipient a couple of minutes to come around, and then ask her to sit up slowly. It is very likely that your client will say that she is "walking on air." Offer your client a cup of water, and tell her to drink some water or at the very least some weak herbal tea when she gets home.

Wash your hands immediately.

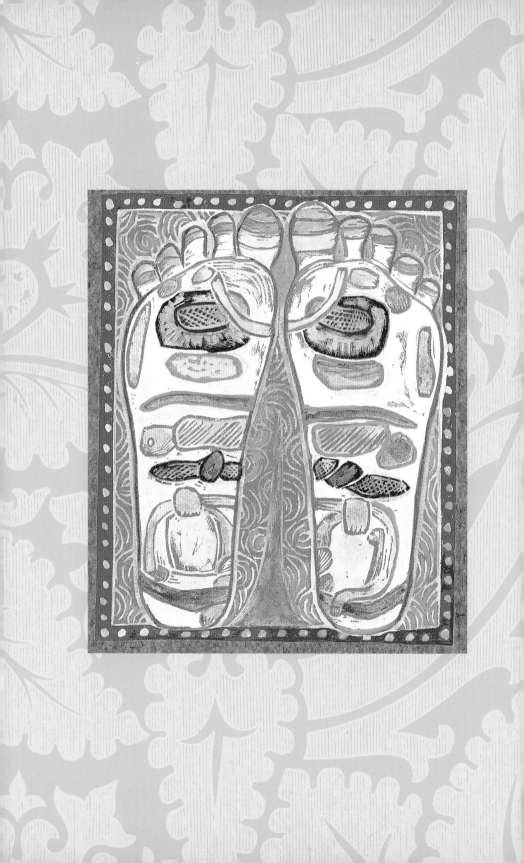

13

SELF-HELP AND ESSENTIAL OILS

THE FIVE-MINUTE MINI-BREAK

Most of us sit at our desks or in front of our computers without a break for far too long. Our necks and shoulders tense up, and soon the muscles begin to ache; we become engrossed in our work and forget to drink something hydrating, and as time goes on we get eye strain and begin to develop a headache or neck pain. Here is a good self-help idea:

- Get up and stretch for two minutes.
- Use the caterpillar walk on the reflexes of the spine on your own hands for two minutes.
- Take a minute to get some water or herbal tea without milk or sugar.

Do this on a regular basis throughout the day. You will feel so much better and be so much more productive.

STUCK IN A TRAFFIC JAM?

Being stuck in traffic is becoming more common these days. It can mean huge amounts of stress as the clock ticks by; you can feel yourself tensing up, and you can begin to feel your heart beat faster. You are late for that appointment and getting later by the second. Now picture this: Instead of concentrating on the clock ticking by, focus on your hands and do your spine reflexes several times. After all, whether you

focus on the traffic and drive yourself crazy or not, the traffic won't move any faster; only your pulse will. So anytime
you feel your blood pressure rising (so to speak), stop and
concentrate on working on your hands. The traffic will move
in no time, and you will feel better.

SHOU—XING (BALLS OF ETERNAL HEALTH)

The Chinese shou-xing balls were created five hundred years
ago during the Ming dynasty. *Shou-xing* means "eternal
health." The emperor's physician had advised him that in order
to treat his failing health he would need to exercise all his vital
organs and at the same time reduce his hypertension. The
balls of eternal health were made to help the emperor get
better. Since then, generation after generation has benefited
from the practice. How do shou-xing balls work?

According to Chinese traditional medicine, which includes
healing therapies to the hands, the eight fingers, two
thumbs, and palms are connected to all the vital organs of
the body. Manipulating the shou-xing balls stimulates vari-
ous reflexes and acupuncture points on the hands, resulting
in an increase in the flow of vital energy and blood in the
body. It promotes muscular tone and bone strength, while
relaxing the mind. It can prevent or reduce hypertension and
stress. Daily exercise with shou-xing balls can increase concentration, promote memory, reduce fatigue and anxiety,
and ultimately extend our lives.

The balls come as a pair, and in different sizes; the pair you choose depends on the size of your hands. Place both balls in the palm of one hand. Using the fingers of that hand, rotate the balls around each other in your palm for five minutes, then change to your other hand.

If the five-minute mini-break does not appeal to you, especially if you are working in a busy office where stretching would attract too much attention, then using the shou-xing balls for five minutes would be a good alternative.

A TOUCH OF AROMATIC LUXURY

You can use aromatherapy essential oils either at the end of a reflexology treatment or for a foot massage. When you don't have time to do a reflexology treatment but have a few minutes to spare for yourself or someone else, this is bliss. The soles of the feet are highly absorbent and will readily absorb the therapeutic properties of essential oils. In general it takes up to twenty minutes for the essentials oils' therapeutic properties to be absorbed by the body through the skin into the bloodstream, where they will remain for seven hours or more.

These compounds can affect pain, inflammation, digestion, and the functioning of the immune system. They can act as powerful antioxidants and so much more. The aromas of these oils can play an important part in the healing process, as they have a direct effect on the brain via the nose.

Warming essential oils in a burner will create a healing space for you to work in.

Essential oils are distilled from plants and are highly concentrated and very strong. For this reason they *must* be diluted in what is known as a "carrier" oil, body lotion, cream, shampoo, or bathwater. Common carrier oils include coconut oil, cocoa butter, olive oil, walnut oil, and almond oil—cold-pressed and organic, if possible.

In theory, there are two exceptions. Lavender oil and tea tree oil are essential oils that can be used undiluted, but you should still exercise caution. However, it is important that you never use these two oils undiluted on children. Although it is safe to use tea tree oil undiluted on adults, it can sting a little, so I would suggest diluting it with a little carrier oil as well.

Essential oils come in three categories, known as "notes":

- The "top notes" are oils that are generally light, and these are the most stimulating and energizing of the oils. Their quality is intense, and they evaporate quickly. These include eucalyptus, peppermint, and lemon.
- The "middle notes" are oils that are strong and potent but not as stimulating as the top notes. These are tea tree, rosemary, geranium, lavender, and chamomile. You will detect these notes in a blend after the top notes have worn off.
- The "base notes" linger longer than the other two, as they evaporate slowly. These are rich, full-bodied, and

heavy. In a blend, you will detect the aroma of the base notes after the others. Two common base notes are clove and sandalwood.

Following are my top ten favorites of the most popular reasonably priced essential oils. These essential oils can be used in conjunction with reflexology, but only in an oil burner rather than on a client's skin. Always buy one hundred percent pure essential oil.

1. TEA TREE

Tea tree is my favorite, but only just, as lavender is a very close second. Tea tree is a natural antifungal oil, which is good for treating all sorts of fungal infections, including vaginal yeast infections, jock itch, athlete's foot, candida, and ringworm. It also helps to boost the immune system; it's a first-aid kit in one little bottle. Tea tree is an antiseptic that you can use to treat minor burns, along with acne, dandruff, cuts, eczema, and scabies. Tea tree oil soothes and calms skin irritations, rashes, and warts and can help to curb the proliferation of some viruses. Tea tree oil is also one of the few aromatherapy oils that may be used undiluted on the skin. It is nontoxic and nonirritating, but it is always advisable to test the skin for sensitivity (if using undiluted) by placing just a tiny amount on the skin. Be prepared to wash it off immediately if there is any sensitivity. A few drops of the undiluted oil may be used for the treatment of athlete's foot, cold sores, cuts, burns, and ringworm infections. It can help reduce pain, and it can promote healing. Some people have found it to be a good insect repellent. Tea tree oil blends well with eucalyptus, lavender, lemon, and rosemary.

2. LAVENDER

I put lavender in second place, but only just. This essential oil can be used for headaches, migraines, burns, wounds, bruises, insect bites, oily skin, acne, eczema, and swellings, as well as for calming insomnia and for mild depression. It is known for its relaxing qualities, and it is helpful in the treatment of inflammation and pain. Put directly on minor burns, this oil instantly relieves the pain. Lavender oil eases tension, fatigue, and feelings of depression. Lavender is relaxing, antiseptic, antibacterial, antidepressant, decongestant, detoxifying, diuretic, and restorative. Lavender oil blends well with eucalyptus, geranium, and lemon.

3. EUCALYPTUS

Eucalyptus has astringent properties that reduce mucous membrane inflammation of the upper respiratory tract. Eucalyptol is the chemical component found in this oil that helps to improve breathing. Earaches can also be treated with eucalyptus. When inhaled, this oil opens up the Eustachian tubes; it drains fluids and relieves pressure, improving hearing and breathing. Eucalyptus is an effective remedy for asthma, bronchitis, sinusitis, whooping cough, and colds. Rubbed onto the skin, eucalyptus oil stimulates blood flow and generates the sensation of warmth, helping to soothe the underlying pain and discomfort of arthritis or muscle aches. It can be used to treat insect bites, and a couple of drops can be added to water and used as a mouthwash. It is often used for household cleaning and in the laundry. Always dilute this oil before using it. Eucalyptus oil blends well with lavender, lemon, and tea tree.

4. PEPPERMINT

Peppermint is good for treating headaches, muscle aches, and digestive disorders such as slow digestion, indigestion, irritable bowel syndrome, nausea, vomiting, and flatulence. Peppermint oil can calm children's recurrent abdominal pains. It helps to relieve the symptoms of a cold, muscular aches and pains, and neuralgia. Always dilute this oil before using it. Peppermint oil blends well with chamomile, eucalyptus, lavender, and rosemary.

5. ROSEMARY

Rosemary is useful for physical and mental fatigue, respiratory problems, asthma, and rheumatic aches and pains. Rosemary oil helps to clear the mind and improve the memory and is an effective treatment for muscular pain and arthritic conditions. It stimulates the circulation, as well as being an excellent detoxifying oil. Always dilute this oil before using it. Rosemary oil blends well with lavender, lemon, and peppermint.

CAUTION Rosemary should be avoided if you are pregnant or have high blood pressure or suffer from epilepsy.

6. LEMON

The aroma of lemon oil increases both concentration and awareness. Some research has shown that when lemon essential oil is diffused throughout a busy office, the staff makes fewer mistakes. Lemon oil helps with cellulite by improving circulation, and it supports the elimination of wastes. It has an affinity with our major detoxification organ, the liver. Lemon oil assists with the exfoliation of dead skin and helps improve the complexion. It is antiseptic and antibacterial and serves as a physical and mental stimulant, a skin tonic, and a circulatory stimulant. It is refreshing, and it enhances the immune system. It gives a clean, fresh feeling. Always dilute this oil before using it. Lemon oil blends well with lavender, sandalwood, geranium, eucalyptus, and rosemary.

CAUTION Lemon oil is phototoxic, which means after using it you can't expose your skin to direct sunlight for six hours.

7. CLOVE

Clove oil is warming and stimulating and has pain-relieving and antiseptic properties. You can soak a cotton ball and swab your gums for quick pain relief from toothache that will serve until you can get to a dentist. Diluted in a carrier oil or lotion, clove oil can numb the pain of arthritis, rheumatism, and sore muscles. Clove oil blends well with lemon and lavender.

> CAUTION! **Use clove oil in moderation, and always dilute it well, using concentrations of no more than two percent to prevent skin irritation (unless you are using it on your gums for toothache). If you have sensitive skin, use clove oil with care.**

8. GERANIUM

Geranium oil is helpful for cuts, sores, and insect bites and as an insect repellent. It soothes skin problems and is useful as an antidepressant, muscle relaxant, and balance for female hormones. Geranium is especially good for oily and dull skin, as it stimulates both the lymphatic and circulatory systems. It is antiseptic, fungicidal, cleansing, and mildly pain relieving, and it reduces inflammation and stops bleeding. Geranium can help acne, bruises, burns, cuts, broken capillaries, varicose veins, dermatitis, cellulite, eczema, ulcers, and wounds. Always dilute this oil before using it. Geranium oil blends well with lemon, lavender, and sandalwood.

9. CHAMOMILE

Chamomile oil is a soothing, gentle relaxant that has been shown to work for a variety of complaints from stress to menstrual cramps. Chamomile has been used for more than two thousand years as a natural treatment for nervous conditions and insomnia. Chamomile oil can be used as a pain reliever for muscle aches and pains, rheumatism, headaches, migraine, neuralgia, toothache, and earache. Chamomile oil can be used for skin problems, including acne, eczema, rashes, wounds, dermatitis, dry, itchy skin, and allergic conditions in general. Always dilute this oil before using it. Chamomile oil blends well with lavender, geranium, and lemon.

10. SANDALWOOD

Sandalwood is deeply tranquil. It stimulates the pineal gland, located in the brain, which is the center of our emotions. Sandalwood can clear and pacify the mind, calm an overheated body, and reduce hyperactivity. Sandalwood can instill a sense of inner peace. It can be beneficial for dry skin, and it supports the nervous and circulatory systems. Always dilute this oil before using it. Sandalwood oil blends with lavender and geranium.

A WORD ABOUT WATER

Clearly, water is neither an oil or an essence, but this liquid is essential for hydration, and most of us don't drink enough of it. We should drink six to eight glasses of water a day for good health. As long as the tap water in your area is clean and pleasant to drink, that's the best choice of water to imbibe, but if you live in an area where it tastes of bleach or chemicals, you might prefer to drink bottled water. If so, choose a brand that doesn't have to travel far so that you minimize the carbon footprint.

conclusion

After reading this book, you might decide to find a qualified practitioner to have regular reflexology treatments. Generally, you need six treatments, spread over a period of six weeks; then you have follow-up treatments, which you can have from once a week to once a month, depending on your health goals and your pocket. Some of you will decide after learning and doing some reflexology at home that you want to become fully qualified reflexologists. Reflexology courses are usually designed to fit around people's jobs, so they are often on weekends. It takes about a year to complete a course, and there is a written and a practical exam at the end of the course. Many of you will use this book to teach yourselves how to treat yourselves and your loved ones. Learning reflexology is a lot of fun, and giving or receiving a treatment can be extremely rewarding. With a little practice you can help to keep yourself, your family, and your friends healthy and happy.

A popular practice in the United States is to have an "exercise buddy" or a "diet buddy," and this has been shown to work well, so I suggest you find a "reflexology buddy," because it's so much more fun if you find a like-minded friend with whom to share this journey of discovery. Even if you decide you don't need a professional treatment yourself, it's a good idea to see a qualified reflexologist for just one treatment session to experience the caterpillar walk. When I was studying alternative treatments, my tutor advised me to find out what the treatments that I give others feel like from the client's perspective, and it was a useful exercise. In this case, it's only fair to tell the reflexologist the purpose of your visit. I am sure he or she would be only too happy to assist you and give you some advice. After all, that is why they took up the practice in the first place—to help others. When you want to train yourself, contact the reflexology associations in your country and ask for a list of accredited practitioners and teachers in your area.

Health magazines carry advertisements from qualified reflexologists. Look for Web sites for reflexology organizations and associations in your area. Word of mouth can be a very good way of finding a practitioner. Contact schools that offer continuing education in your area, as they may have students who are looking for feet to experiment on. Look in your local newspaper.

Whatever path you choose, have fun!

index

31901050567736